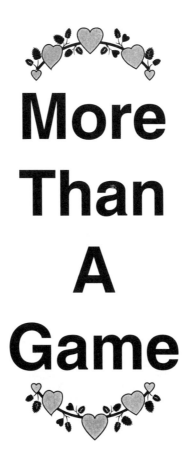

More
Than
A
Game

A New Focus on Senior Activity Services

by Brenda Corbett, C.T.R.S.

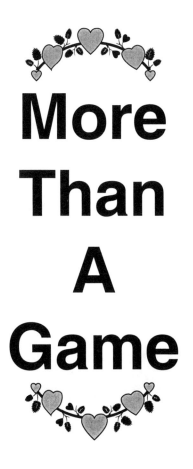

More Than A Game

A New Focus on Senior Activity Services

by Brenda Corbett, C.T.R.S.

Venture Publishing, Inc.
1999 Cato Avenue, State College, PA 16801

Production Manager: Richard Yocum
Manuscript Editing and Design: Michele L. Barbin
Additional Editing: Matthew S. Weaver and Diane K. Bierly
Cover Design: Sandra Sikorski, Sikorski Design

Library of Congress Catalogue Card Number 97-80848
ISBN 0-910251-94-0

To Karl and Dani,
For your unconditional love.

Special thanks to Peter and Sheila Hutt, illustrators
for this book, my parents and biggest supporters.

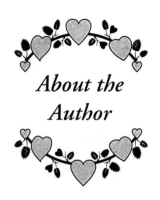

About the Author

Brenda Corbett has dedicated almost twenty years to the service of older adults. A native of Canada, she earned her degree in Therapeutic Recreation from the University of Waterloo in Ontario.

Corbett first found her calling to long-term care at Rockway Gardens Senior Center in Kitchener, Ontario. She has directed activity services at a full range of facilities: retirement communities, assisted living facilities, nursing homes, continuing care retirement communities and adult day-care centers. Her professional journey has taken her to facilities in Canada and positions in Arizona, Florida, North Carolina, and Ohio.

Creativity and conscientiousness are the keys to her success with older adults and with her staff. This, her first book, shares those keys with activity professionals. Corbett has developed dozens of innovative programs over the years.

Her latest project has her directing the efforts of Trinity Foundation International, a foundation dedicated specifically to the elderly in long-term care settings.

Brenda lives in Cincinnati with her husband, Karl, and three children: Dani, Nora and Dan.

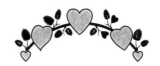

Contents

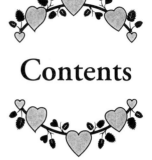

Contents

In the abstracts of the author's experiences, the names of the individuals mentioned, both living and deceased, have been changed to protect the confidentiality of the residents. These asides are intended to be inspirational to practitioners, and encourage innovation and creativity in meeting the needs of residents.

No More Bingo!

Martha was a resident with dementia. She could talk to a degree, but Martha had difficulty understanding and being understood. Martha loved to be with people. She would make conversation with anyone who had time to sit and listen. Martha walked all over our facility, and greeted all the residents and all the visitors. One day, I gave her an "authentic" facility nametag with her name and the words "Resident Greeter" underneath. She was in heaven. Martha wore her nametag with pride and honor. I asked her to stand by the door and welcome people. She was a natural. She was able to tell visitors where the reception desk was and say, "Hi, how are you?" over 50 times a day. If she ever misplaced her nametag she felt lost and without a purpose. With her nametag and her "official" status, Martha felt important, needed and loved. All residents have a genuine need to be connected to someone or something.

The most challenging part of working in a nursing home is the difficulty involved in connecting with many residents. Residents who can tell you their pleasures, needs and complaints are easy to deal with, because you can communicate and understand each other. Whether or not the communication is positive, it is at least taking place, and can thus be addressed. On the other hand, the residents with little or no ability to speak cannot always have their needs met. There is a gulf between these residents and their caregivers. This gulf can be bridged only if the caregiver is willing to accept the residents, and work with them on whatever level they are currently functioning. With this acceptance, relationships can be formed. With understanding, you can create a loving and comfortable home for the residents. Establishing relationships is the key to creating quality of life in a nursing home.

Residents are not just the reason for the nursing home—they *are* the nursing home. No other reason exists to maintain a nursing home except the people who live there. This seems obvious, but needs to be fully understood. Nursing homes care for a group of people who are not able to manage on their own. Beyond that, not many generalities apply. Summarizing needs and creating programs for a resident population is not a simple exercise because of the unique backgrounds, needs and abilities of each resident involved.

This is where a specialized activity services department comes in. It is the responsibility of the activity services department to correctly assess and understand each resident. This includes his or her strengths, weaknesses, and his or her potential to participate in therapeutic activities. Activity services must also educate and orient all the facility's staff in understanding all levels of cognitive ability. In understanding, a staff member accepts and fulfills his or her role as an effective caregiver and supporter. Of course, activity services personnel must lead the way by example, patiently accepting and providing suitable activities for all levels of cognitive ability.

Selection of activities must be presented for the current residents in a facility. No two facilities' activity services can be the same because the residents they provide for are not the same. Plan, program and implement for each unique group of residents. Whatever a resident's abilities and problems might be, each resident deserves attention and respect. Respect does not mean simply offering daily programming to "use" their time. A day can be very long for a nursing home resident, but residents deserve more than simple programming to fill their days. Granted, there is some value in "time fillers." But, residents need programs created and designed to suit their individual needs, their current abilities, and their former lifestyles.

Through a variety of specific activities, the activity services department can help overcome many of the stereotypes about residents who are cognitively impaired. The activities that are organized are simply a means to an end. Activities are the most critical component in the relationship between the facility and the residents. The residents must feel as though they are the center of the universe. Activity services professionals are their connection to the world.

The key to successful programs lies in providing activities that make sense to every resident and to every employee in the facility. Employees need to understand the importance of activities. They must witness activities making a difference in the lives of the residents. Life is easier for other departments when residents are busy, and when they are interested in the programs the facility offers. The more satisfying a life you create for your residents, the less likely it is that they will have complaints and problems. From the nurse's aides and housekeepers to the nursing supervisor, the more the staff understands the purpose and goals of the activities program, the more cooperation the activities services department will get toward making programs work for the residents.

All nursing homes have bingo and special events, such as entertainment from the community. These diversionary programs have great merit. There are many residents who enjoy bingo and enjoy being entertained. The positive aspects of bingo are many. It offers the resident more opportunity to be independent and in control than most other activities. Bingo is a self-directed activity in a group setting. For the individual who does not want to associate too much with other residents, this is the perfect way to be part of the community. Bingo is rewarding for the residents who have enjoyed this game for many years. They know the rules and are very confident that this is something at which they can be successful.

Bingo is easy. For all the residents who live in a nursing home, this is one game that needs no explanation. It is easy even for the resident who has lost some cognitive ability. It makes for a very positive situation with very little to lose. Bingo is an outlet for people who have spent their lives betting and gambling. This allows them to continue their lifestyle. Bingo allows participants to be financially independent. The money is not much, but it is all theirs, with no strings attached. The game is competitive without putting pressure on anyone. It is a sedentary game with a personal competitive side. It allows the players to "get away" for an hour. Bingo is universal. No matter what background, religion or life experience, everyone can play.

Diversionary programs such as bingo and entertainment from the community are a necessary and vital part of the activities offered at a nursing home. But, they are the only activities offered at many nursing homes. If that is all an activity services department has to offer, there is much room for improvement. Diversionary programs are a very small part of what makes life for a resident both worthwhile and enjoyable. It doesn't matter how you look at it, it is imperative that your activity program offers more. If an activity program relies entirely on bingo, games, and entertainment from the community, then the department is still living in the past. This is no longer acceptable programming for any nursing facility.

Chapter One

The biggest complaint about bingo and games is that many residents are not able to play or have absolutely no interest in playing. What happens to the resident who is piling one bingo chip on top of another? Instinct (education) tells us to approach the resident and correct him or her, to help him or her put the chips on the correct number. The activity staff have a need for residents to play the game correctly. This is true for the resident who is interested in winning the game, but not true for the "stacker." It should be quite apparent that these residents either have no interest in the game, or even ability to follow the rules.

This is a perfect example of why bingo cannot be the centerpiece of the programming in the activity department. It is a successful event with a number of residents. But what about residents who are not in the least bit interested? What about the resident who cannot understand the caller? How does a resident who cannot hear manage to participate? What about the resident who cannot see the card to cover the numbers? What about the resident who cries out and interrupts the game? What do you do with the resident who bursts out in song in the middle of a game? What about the resident who has hated bingo all his or her life? What about a resident's moral objection to gambling or a simple aversion to the game?

Entertainment and diversion are necessary, but cannot fulfill the variety of needs found in a nursing facility's population. Many residents cannot enjoy games and entertainment. With the information provided in this book, you can reach those residents, too. The population of nursing home residents has changed dramatically in the past few years. Remember when many residents came to a facility because they wanted company or needed help with daily routines? These residents were old and did not have anyone to care for them.

Due to soaring costs of healthcare, people now stay outside the nursing home for as long as they can. Today's residents have no alternative except nursing home placement. There is often a triggering experience that brings a resident into a nursing home. This could be anything from breaking a hip to being found in a potentially dangerous situation or environment. These people are not able to care for themselves. Some are on restrictive diets. Some are unable to control their bowels and bladder. No one is available to help them to the extent that is needed for them to remain at home. They have become cognitively unable to make appropriate decisions that used to be very simple for them. As a result of these circumstances, today's residents are less likely to be alert, aware and oriented. That's why therapeutic activities are so necessary. Activity services are dealing with a different type of resident. We cannot ignore these residents, so we must develop new avenues to reach them.

Activity professionals are responsible for the well-being of the residents. Indeed, there are other disciplines involved in daily care, but the activity staff becomes the residents' new family. Activity services personnel are the center of the day-to-day existence of the elderly in the nursing home. A major key to using this book successfully is understanding each resident well enough to know which techniques to apply. Activity services professionals spend time with residents on a consistent basis for a variety of purposes. As a result, they understand the personalities, the likes, and dislikes of each individual. Activity professionals should strive toward the following goal:

Every resident can be part of the community and enjoy the rest of his or her life within his or her personal limits.

This book is about how to provide the quality of life to which every resident is entitled.

The groups in this book are here to start you thinking about the limitless possibilities available to you and your department. These groups are described in detail to start you on the road to a successful, productive activity services department. Potentially, there is no end to what you can create and design, based on the concepts behind these groups. With dedication and creativity, you can create spectacular activity programs driven by a dynamic and caring staff.

There are some things you must remember once this book is put away and you begin implementing these programs. Your number one priority is to make sure you reach every resident in your facility. This means that no resident is left alone or falls between the cracks. Whether you are working in a facility of 50 or 500, your mission is the same. All residents must be treated as individuals and permitted the opportunity to participate in their activity of preference. Treat your activity services staff with respect. Remember, what you get from your staff will only meet the level of expectation you put on them.

Do not be disappointed if a program does not work. Everyone is learning, and sometimes failure allows you to grow and enables you to develop the kinds of programs that will be successful and profound in your facility.

Activities are changing by the minute in the long-term care business. With the increase in population of older adults, activities no longer can afford to take a backseat. Change yesterday's thought patterns, and accept responsibility to maintain or improve the cognitive, physical, spiritual and emotional well-being of your residents. This means more than simply changing the calendar of events. It involves changing your mission as a department and your vision as a professional. You must feel it and live it day-to-day in your facility.

Chapter One

This aging population is a continuously changing population. These changes directly relate to your department. As a true professional, you must constantly educate yourself in order to keep up with the changes. What kind of person will be coming into your facility? How much has the average resident changed from five years ago? From ten years ago? Know the people you serve—have the will to serve them. This book is dedicated to developing your skills and encouraging your will to serve.

The following terms and definitions are used throughout this text:

Therapeutic groups is a term that is new to the field of activity services. It summarizes the marriage between activities and therapy. It also describes activity programs in a way that helps explain their value to a facility.

Intimacy is a term used to describe the immediate moment you have connected and shared with a resident: the here and now, the eye contact, the present involvement and "communication" happening at that time.

Activity services department is a new and innovative term which every activity professional should start using. This term is designed to inform others that activity staff wears many hats. They are involved with the resident as an individual and within the group settings they provide. They handle mandated paperwork. They help both the families of residents and the community as a whole. It describes the contemporary role in assisted living, retirement communities, subacute units, and long-term care facilities. *Activity therapy department*, another term coined recently to describe the profession, stagnates the department by not explaining all areas of the department's involvement. It has a limited, clinical, and rather mundane sound.

Another new and clinical-sounding descriptor is the word *patient* to describe nursing home residents. The managed care phenomenon is bringing hospital terminology into the nursing home. Patients do not reside at a hospital. Patients stay in hospitals for brief periods. Avoid this "new" terminology. Until nursing homes are called nursing hospitals, residents should not be called patients.

Innovation and Evaluation

2

Building therapeutic groups around the residents is only part of the equation of good programming. Programming a full and comprehensive calendar of events is vital for a fully functioning department. Therapeutic groups are a vital component in a perfect activity department.

Here's a "full month" outline that I have used for almost twenty years that I have been in this business. Measure your program plan against this benchmark. It has helped me create innovative and exciting programs month after month:

20	exercise programs—including walking
20	therapeutic groups (or more depending on number of staff)
over 20	volunteering opportunities
12	mind-based games—including bingo
10	room visits
10	active games
10	religious programs—all denominations
8 to 10	evening programs
4	food carts
4	resident meetings (e.g., resident council, food committee meeting)
3 or 4	outings (or as many as transportation capabilities permit)
4	arts and crafts programs
4	baking programs
4	men's events
4	women's events
4	movies
2	associate/staff involvement events (e.g., baking contests, chili cook-off)

> 1 birthday party
> 1 special event
> 1 *new* entertainment
> 1 *new* activity

These numbers are based on one month. The "new activity" and "new entertainment" have been a good philosophy to keep momentum going. Don't be afraid to discontinue an unsuccessful activity. This is not a reflection on your abilities, but on the interests of the residents. Change, grow and adapt to your residents, their lifestyles, and their interests. Stay innovative! Some of these activities can overlap, such as volunteer programs and women's programs, or movies and evening programs.

Remember When You Create Your Calendar:

1. **Be creative, try things out.** The worst that can happen is that the day or program is not successful. When that happens, be willing to say you won't offer that program again.

   Example: Wear your favorite M&M color. Most of my staff argued that it would never work, but every employee in the entire facility dressed up. The discussion and fun that took place was spontaneous and exciting for everyone.

2. **Allow the entire staff of the facility to be part of your creative force.** Create committees, or use the suggestions of the associates for event ideas.

   Example: A nursing supervisor recommended having "Purple Day"—everyone dressed in the color purple. We called it "International Purple Day" as if this had been going on for years, all over the world.

3. **Themes have always proven to be successful.** This allows you to follow a concept or idea throughout the whole day and it almost creates the event itself.

   Example: Purple Day continued throughout the day with a showing of *The Color Purple* and serving chips, purple dip and cranberry cocktails at Happy Hour.

4. **Inform the public.** When you have an event or when staff are dressed for a special theme day, post a message in the front lobby informing visitors and families of your theme, and the different outfits they might encounter during their visit.

5. **Can you include the community in some way?** Ask this question about each special event. Community involvement gives your department needed recognition. You can create great (and *free*) publicity for your facility, too.

Example: The facility had a special Thanksgiving dinner for the residents. We asked a high-school basketball team to come as volunteers to help serve the residents and move tables. It was even more memorable when the basketball team members all showed up in tuxedos.

6. **Keep communication open with the food services department.** They are a very important part of a successful calendar. Food should be used in constructive and innovative ways. I have seen great responses from food carts (explained in The Work Group, chapter four) that offer various foods to the residents on a weekly basis.

Example: Seasonal favorite foods have always been popular— for example, serve pumpkin pie in the fall or strawberry short-cake in the summer. We even tried a pickle cart for Oktoberfest and it was a smashing success. The residents rarely get the opportunity to eat dill pickles!

7. **Delegate responsibility to your staff.** You cannot do everything yourself, and that is not your purpose as a director. Failure can be a learning experience in this business. Give your staff full responsibility for an event. Make sure your expectations of the event are clear before you start this process. Let them take the event from the conception to its implementation in front of the residents and staff. Be there to help, but let the decisions come from the coordinators. Have your staff complete an evaluation (see page 11) after each event. I recommend that you and the coordinator of the event complete the form separately and then get together to discuss it. This provides a perfect

opportunity for open communication and positive feedback. Make sure the negative comments are discussed thoroughly, along with ideas for improvement.

8. **Rule of thumb—Remember to offer seven programs per day including room visits.** A typical day could look like this on your calendar:

9:00 a.m.	Coffee Time
10:00 a.m.	A Touching Moment
10:30 a.m.	Mind Boggler
11:00 a.m.	Name Game
2:00 p.m.	Musical Entertainment with the "Swingers"
3:30 p.m.	Hospitality Club
7:00 p.m.	Bible Study

9. **One resident, one day at a time.** Find a niche for each resident and you're on the right track. All your residents need is the empowerment and self-esteem we are trying to help them achieve in this—their new home.

Program Evaluation

Name of Program: _____

Date of Program: _____ Number in Attendance: _____

Staff in Attendance: _____

Music? If yes, who: _____

Location: _____

Positive Aspects of Program: _____

_____

_____

_____

_____

Negative Aspects of Program: _____

_____

_____

_____

_____

Any Other Comments:

_____

_____

_____

_____

_____

_____

Therapeutic Recreation in Long-Term Care

3

"So, what's the point? She's not going to get any better, you know." The words hung like a dark cloud in the room. Terry was bringing her mother to stay in our facility. I had just finished telling her what my activity staff might do to help her mother fit in, and feel at home. Somehow, my hope and enthusiasm were just not making an impression on Terry. I started over. "Terry, the activities we plan for your Mom are more than just fun and games. We really try to reach people, and help them reach out to others. I don't know if she'll get better or not. I do know we can make her life better while she is here with us. I won't let this place become a warehouse for your mother, or for anyone else."

Therapy is best defined as *the process of treating and caring for someone in order to combat disease, injury or mental distress.* The word therapy is used throughout the rest of this book with that definition in mind. Therapy is commonly used to describe medical activity, nutritional plans, and the formal disciplines of mental health. It is very appropriate, though, to describe the work of the activity professional as therapy.

Recreation therapy is the use of leisure time and leisure pursuits as a form of treatment. In the nursing home, the activity services department makes use of residents' time not spent in activities of daily living (ADL). These ADLs include personal care from nurse's aides, the taking of medications, bathing, eating, and everything else necessary to maintain physical functioning. Activity services takes it from there. Activity professionals are involved in the social, emotional, spiritual and educational well-being of the resident.

Activity professionals provide *treatment or care directed toward healing*. Treatment and caring is the heart of recreation therapy, and the main focus of this book. Involving residents in activities and recreation creates therapy at an individual, personal level. The purpose behind every activity described in this book is the enhancement of quality of life. With these programs, you can help make life in the nursing home better for residents of all conditions and abilities.

"She's not going to get better, you know." That's hard to accept sometimes, but the nursing home is not usually a stepping stone for recuperation. Nursing home residents must live with their conditions. They seldom are able to leave the nursing home environment. Maintenance is a very acceptable goal for programs in activity services. It must be stressed that maintenance, in itself, is an accomplishment.

We will eventually discuss therapeutic programs in subacute care. Those programs are designed to be rehabilitative and can be altered to fit short-term residents. Participating in therapeutic programs will help channel the rehabilitation potential of these short-term residents. Retirement communities and assisted living facilities (ALFs) are also discussed, and appropriate programs are recommended for this population in chapter eight.

The key to providing therapy is the understanding that clear goals and objectives must guide all your activities. There must be a purpose to what you are doing with the residents and a standard by which you measure your accomplishments. Do not overemphasize head counts, thereby making residents participate in activities that have no meaning or purpose for them. As activity professionals, we must improve the services we deliver, emphasizing quality rather than quantity.

Applying the term *therapy* to the work of activity services is a new concept. This is a term that medical staff have always "owned." With a growing emphasis on "total care" and residents' quality of life, this will change. Taking ownership of the term *therapy* for our work as activity professionals helps us gain recognition for our important role in long-term care.

Diversionary groups and entertainment are still vital. They are one reason activities services are so important to the resident. But we must step away, at least in part, from the bingo and entertainment business, and apply ourselves more to treatment and care. Therapy is the heart of therapeutic recreation and activities. Once you have used the ideas in this book, you will find that the purpose of your "fun and games" will have changed for both you and your residents. Once the "therapy" concept is applied to your activity services department, your efforts will command more respect from other department heads. The department will be more visible to administration. Your staff and your residents will benefit while fun and enjoyment fill the hall of your facility.

With these goals and benefits in mind, you are ready to study the notion of *therapeutic programs* conducted by activity services. The ideal way to apply recreation therapy in the activity services department is to implement therapeutic programs. This term describes treatment or care for residents in a group setting. This book will describe dozens of group activities you can start using right away. These descriptions will talk about the "why" as well as the "how-to." Each therapeutic program is designed for a specific audience with specific purposes and goals.

> *Lee is a sweet lady from the hills of Kentucky. She has two children, but neither one has visited since her admission four years ago. She has always been a quiet woman. Lee can speak, but only very softly. She has some dementia. She is a good observer, but never a participant, no matter what diversionary group she attends. Lee was invited to be part of an interest-based therapeutic group called "Let's Talk Dirt." Her past lifestyle as a farmer in Kentucky allowed her to excel in this gardening group. She is now involved in plant care as much as anyone has ever been in this facility. This is a simple horticulture therapy program, but it is meaningful to Lee. She is no longer just "there," existing for the sake of existing. This small therapeutic group works wonders for Lee by providing a positive successful environment where Lee can find familiarity, comfort and satisfaction.*

Groups work because each one has a purpose, and because members are assessed to make sure they will find benefits and enjoyment.

> *Mildred was socially isolated. She could not make herself understood, nor did she appear to understand others. She was not responsive, but no one really knew what she could (or could not) hear and understand. An initial assessment, completed with the help of her family, showed that Mildred enjoyed music. Our activity services staff would visit her in her room. They would play music, hoping she enjoyed it. Some of them had misgivings. They did not know how to act while alone in a room with an unresponsive resident. This was not contributing to employee morale, and*

certainly was not helping Mildred. So, I brought together a half-dozen residents who enjoyed music—spiritual and gospel music in this case. I assigned staff to bring Mildred in to join the group. Mildred got stimulation from the music. She smiled, and even held the hand of the facilitator. This was more than she had ever done during room visits. She was no longer alone. She was now with other people who had similar interests. Mildred still gets personal attention because the group is so small. One group leader is meeting our goals for Mildred along with six other residents' needs. This simple therapeutic group has accomplished more in one session per week than ten room visits a month had ever done.

Room visits are an important part of activity services department's duties. There are good reasons for room visits, but unless you have an unlimited budget, you cannot meet the demand for room visits with your existing personnel. Assess every resident involved in the room visits and create a profile, asking these questions:

- What are the needs of the residents receiving room visits?

- Is the resident bed-bound by choice or necessity?

- If it is by choice, is the resident's self-imposed isolation due to shyness, lack of trust, or some other factor?

- What is the resident's level of cognitive ability?

- Is he or she verbal?

- Is he or she depressed?

- Has the resident spent much of his or her life alone?

- Does the resident have isolation orders?

- Does his or her family and friends visit regularly? Often? Seldom? Never?

- Is the resident combative or unable to be in a group for some reason?

Assess your "room visit" residents carefully, just as you would an active, participating resident. Find out their interests and their former lifestyle. Involving family members in the assessment is mandatory if the resident cannot give you all the information you need. This assessment data will be the basis for forming new therapeutic groups and assigning residents to existing ones. Therapeutic programs allow the room-visit resident to be in a small group with people who have similar interests. If they are shy and reserved, residents will feel more at ease in a small group. If their interests are assessed accurately and programs implemented properly, then the members' interests are taken into account. They *will* participate.

The resident who is present at activities, but not involved, is being slighted. Residents can be overlooked for a number of reasons. Those with hearing and vision problems might easily be ignored or neglected. Being disruptive can keep a resident out of some activities. An often neglected resident is the shy "loner" who does not make a sound—whether happy or sad. But, there are *no* exceptions as to who participates in therapeutic programs. If a resident fits the criteria for group membership (that could simply be "hard of hearing"), the resident will be invited to participate in that therapeutic group. Each therapeutic group has a goal. Each will have a set of objectives to reach. The result or outcome can be very general and is different for each group.

To get the desired results, the activity professional must understand the goals of a group, who it is designed for, how to run the group successfully, and who should be invited. Each of the groups described in this book have a distinct criteria for participation with filters to help you decide who belongs in each group. It takes time to establish group assignments. There are no shortcuts to this process. If you are really going to provide therapy, you must gather information on every resident. You must understand your groups and goals. You will need to reassess residents regularly. You will have to make sure group leaders understand the concepts involved. As the front-line staff, group leaders should know whether each group assignment is a stepping stone to another group, or simply a maintenance function.

Once you have assigned residents to groups on paper, all you need to do is establish a schedule, guide the group leaders, and make sure residents attend. Preparation for your groups will be the key to total success with your therapeutic programs. You are virtually guaranteed victory. The following chapters will tell you about the kinds of groups you will have the opportunity to set up, and give detailed information about each one.

Low-Functioning Groups

4

We just called her Mary Smith, and I suppose that really was her name. She had a third-grade education and rarely talked. One day, though, she surprised us all. Sitting in a small group, she was asked to identify some common items related to school. For the first time, she was identifying everything correctly. As Mary held the pen, she suddenly motioned that she wanted to write. As soon as she was presented with paper, Mary began to write, scrawling in a childlike hand, two words— Charlotte Smith. We asked, "Who is that?" She answered, "It's me!" As we posed questions to her about this new name, she told us it was the name she preferred to be called. After four years of seeing her every day, we finally found out how Charlotte preferred to be addressed. It was a simple thing, but so important to her. Our activity group, called Connections, had helped us connect with Charlotte in a way nothing else had.

Groups discussed in this chapter—

- Sensations

- Connections

- Trivia Time

- Radio Daze / Movie Mania

- The Work Group

- Light Touch

- The Name Game

- Spell and Tell

The needs of the resident with low cognitive ability will be summarized in this chapter in a general way. This is not entirely fair, as every person is unique and experiences his or her disability differently. But in presenting this concept of therapy and assigning residents to these groups, it is effective. We often deal with people who cannot communicate effectively. They rarely make eye contact, often have trouble hearing, and do not speak well or clearly. These cognitively challenged residents are frequently overlooked in activities planning. What activities really improve the quality of life for residents who can barely speak? Typical games and large group activities are no longer effective in providing quality in their day-to-day lives. The residents with low cognitive ability are often neglected because they are not sociable, and their skills are limited. Staff do not always understand their needs and often do not respond to them as they do the more oriented residents.

The first five therapeutic groups discussed in this chapter are primarily for residents with low cognitive abilities who experience communication impairments, decreasing mental abilities and difficulty communicating their needs on a consistent basis. Whether you are in a room visit or involved in a simple greeting, receiving a response from these residents is an exciting and worthwhile event. Maybe simple eye contact will spark some recognition. Perhaps they just follow your movement with their eyes.

Working to increase social relationships for residents with low cognitive ability is a realistic goal for every therapeutic group. By putting these groups to work, the activity staff establishes a trusting relationship with residents. With trust, you can generate response and involvement. You can help the residents maintain or even improve their skills in a social situation. You are creating an intimacy that the residents do not experience in any other form throughout their day, and throughout their life at the facility. This intimacy can cause remarkable changes in their behavior and their abilities.

Knowing someone cares about you as an individual produces results that sometimes go beyond explanation. Showing that you care as an activity services professional can involve little more than simply being there and facilitating your group with the residents. Your personal involvement will provide the intimacy they need so desperately. Every resident has the right to be treated as an individual. No other attitude is acceptable—from the activity services department or anyone else. The response you get will depend on the individual resident. Activity staff must assess residents accurately and communicate with each other effectively, so they will know what to expect from each resident.

Getting right answers or correct responses is not as important as creating connections. Connections can take place between a group's facilitator and a resident, between a resident and his or her surroundings, and between residents. In a group setting, it is amazing how successful a resident feels when he or she participates in any way. But it must be stressed to the activity services staff that the goal of these groups is not to elicit "correct" responses. This important piece of information helps create more realistic goals for residents, and establishes a structured environment for their personal version of success.

The following nine therapeutic groups are for the lower functioning resident. Some of these titles will give you a good idea of what happens in these groups. This chapter discusses Sensations, Connections, Trivia Time, Radio Daze, Movie Mania, The Work Group, Light Touch, The Name Game, and Spell and Tell.

Criteria for participation in these low-functioning groups are very broad. Look only for the level of cognition:

- Little or no ability to understand or be understood—ability is limited to making concrete requests, responds sometimes to simple, direct communication;

- Little or no decision-making ability—decisions are poor and cues and supervision are required;

- Little or no ability to verbalize—episodes of incoherent or unclear speech;

- Short attention span—little or no ability to focus on one topic;

Chapter Four

- Cognitive ability varies over the course of the day; and

- Does not recall events after five minutes—short-term memory problems.

Sensations

This group is for the resident with very low cognitive ability. Sensations helps residents use all of their senses to identify common items. Being able to verbally communicate is not a requirement for this group. The residents do not need full use of all five senses. They can be successful with only one.

Goal: To provide an intimate setting for identifying a certain object.

Objectives:

- Provide a social setting to combat the isolation many residents experience;

- Provide an opportunity to stimulate all five senses during one group meeting;

- Encourage participants to use long-term memory to help recall the object; and

- Encourage use of all social skills to communicate answers.

Sensations is directed at residents who do not participate successfully in diversionary groups. These are the residents that, for one reason or another, have no success in large groups. The residents who are involved in this therapeutic group often miss out on other activities because the activity services staff feel they will not "get anything" from them. Sensations can be much more effective than room visits because of the socialization involved. With this activity, residents have a chance to be part of a group environment—a chance they might not get otherwise. Members must be carefully screened since the simplicity of the group could offend some residents.

Group Content and Setup

This therapeutic group is based on the five senses. It stimulates every sense while providing an opportunity for the resident to successfully identify common objects. The primary focus of this group is to socialize and be in direct contact with a staff member. You will find membership in Sensations to be very stable. Changes in the group occur when a resident dies or is moved to a new facility.

Chapter Four

Harvey was in the last stage of Alzheimer's. He no longer received visitors. His family felt it was no use to come because he couldn't communicate appropriately with them. Harvey was placed in a Sensations group. The first item Harvey was asked to identify was coffee. His facilitator had a cup of coffee, coffee grounds, and a picture of a cup of coffee. Harvey had his eyes closed most of the time during group, but every once in a while would make eye contact. Our facilitator gave him a taste of the coffee. She helped him sip the coffee and waited. He turned to her and looked directly in her eyes and asked, "Where's my paper?" This was the first time Harvey had spoken in months.

Your choice of items for Sensations can be quite diverse, and you can use more than one prop for each item. The important thing is to stimulate all five senses when identifying each item. You will begin by introducing an item you have selected without mentioning its name. Often, the voice of the facilitator is the hearing stimulation part of the group's activity. Make sure you do not choose items or sounds that can be confused with other words.

The facilitator welcomes everyone, just as in most groups, but very specifically addresses each resident, introducing himself or herself to the resident and explaining that the residents are participating in Sensations. The facilitator proceeds to stimulate the first sense (order does not matter) and holds the item and discusses the item with the resident without mentioning the name of the item. The group leader discusses the item very directly. The facilitator should use three to six word sentences, like: "What is this?" or "Tell me what you see?" or "What do you think this is?" It is a good idea to repeat questions, but with different phrases. Do not be discouraged with a lack of recognition. There are other senses to work on: "It's good in the morning," "It's good when it's hot," "Do you like it strong?" "I take cream and sugar," and so on. Use your imagination to help each resident distinguish what he or she is experiencing. Continue this process until all the senses have been stimulated.

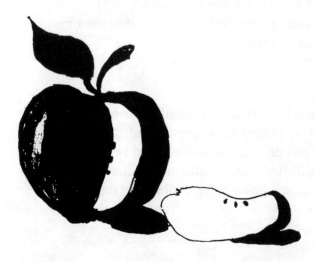

Sensations is an intimate group—intimacy is the key goal of this group. Remember that your purpose is not to get correct answers. You are there to share moments and spend time with the group. You are in a group, but you are experiencing intimate, one-on-one time. The group does not progress at a very fast pace. Of paramount importance is the facilitator's ability to keep the group focused and in the here and now. The present moment is all that matters. This is time devoted entirely to the group members, time when they are important. Below are some themes that have proven to be successful:

Coffee: Coffee in a cup, picture of coffee, sound of a percolator, coffee grounds.

Onions: Sliced up in small amounts, picture of an onion.

Pickles: Closed jar of pickles, pickles (sliced for residents to hold), picture of a pickle.

Lemons: Lemon extract, whole and sliced lemons, picture of a lemon, the song "Lemon Tree" (various artists, notably Peter, Paul and Mary).

Apples: Applesauce, whole and sliced apples, picture of an apple.

Animals: Recordings of the sounds of various animals. Any animal can be used. You can even create the smell of the animal (i.e., bring in hay when discussing a horse). Use lifelike models or toys (i.e., plastic frog), or even just a picture of an animal. Stuffed toys are a poor choice, though, since they are not realistic enough to evoke the desired response.

Make sure you are wearing gloves if you are working with food. Supply enough samples of the food for all the residents since they should not eat anything that was handled by others. Once the group is established, you may want to supply cups and plates marked with the residents' names.

Since the group moves slowly, and involves a lot of one-on-one interaction, limit its size to six to eight residents. This group lasts half an hour. Place the group in a half-circle with the facilitator in an office swivel chair in the center of the circle. Make sure the facilitator has all the props needed for the group prior to the beginning of the group, since leaving to locate props is inappropriate. Place the residents in the same location every time. Their space in the group seems to be very meaningful to them. Over time, they will identify very strongly with the facilitator and the environment. Themes can be used for an entire month. Changes in themes are more to keep the facilitator interested than the residents.

Make sure you stimulate as many senses as possible for each item. Use an item that appeals to at least four of the five senses. Sensations is a one-on-one group activity. Do not become discouraged when one or more participants cannot identify an item. Keep trying. Some residents identify an item after four weeks of the same item. Do not get bored with the residents' apparent inability. Do whatever you can to help the residents succeed. This does make their lives more meaningful.

Connections

Connections provides an opportunity for residents who are verbal (but perhaps confused about time and place) to identify items with which they are familiar. The focus will be to attain participation, and guarantee a level of success that allows residents to experience the pride of accomplishment.

Goal: Provide a stimulating environment to increase socialization and communication with staff and other group members through the use of familiar objects.

Objectives:

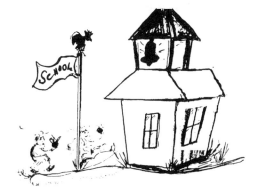

- To identify items;

- To identify the theme of the group of items and form other connections;

- To form interpersonal relationships with other group members; and

- To relate to the facilitator on an intimate level.

Connections encourages the residents to recognize a set of related items. Recognizing these items should bring to mind the purpose of each one. With that, participants can remember and discuss the items, and mentally build relationships between them. They'll use short-term memory to identify and associate the items and their uses. They'll use their long-term memory for recall of their past experience. By examining items in their hands and in the hands of those around them, they are drawn out, to connect with their immediate environment. The interplay between group members is part of the way this group succeeds in reaching its members.

> *"Pass that along to Edna, please," was the facilitator's comment. Edna is able to identify the item herself, and then passes it down the line. She helps Cora hold the item. Across the room Richard speaks out and says, "Let me help you, Cora. It is a piece of jewelry. Still need help? It is a necklace." Richard is beaming, so proud of himself for knowing, and for helping his friends to succeed. Skills like teamwork are built in this group.*

Chapter Four

Group Content and Setup

The list of topics that work in Connections is just about unlimited. For each group topic, it's good to have six to eight items. Here are some themes that have proven to be successful:

School: Chalk, a chalkboard (a small one like the residents might have carried to school), pencil, pen, lunchbox, glue, eraser.

Gardening: Gardening tools (which participants should name), dirt, gardening gloves, a hand shovel/trowel, seeds.

Baking: Spatula, mixing bowls, flour, hand mixer, baking pan, vanilla, baking soda or powder.

Tools: Wrench, hammer, screwdriver, nail, nut and bolt, picture of a saw.

Cooking: Cooking pot or pan, cutting board, tongs, potato masher, serving spoon, cooking oil, spatula.

Beauty: Bobby pins, curlers, brush, comb, mirror, beads, necklaces, hair net, emery board, makeup brush, snood, foundation.

Sewing: A spool of thread, crochet needles, small sewing scissors, tape measure, fabric, a thimble, yarn.

***Wedding:** Bride and groom cake decorations, a garter, lace, rice, wedding pictures, bridal bouquet.

***Babies:** Bib, baby food, diaper (cloth is preferable), rattle, bottle, baby pictures.

---

* **Note:** The topics, wedding and babies, can be very emotional for participants.

Setup for Connections is simple and works the same way every time. This group is easily managed with six to eight participants. It works well if there is one item for each participant. Seat the residents in a half-circle with the facilitator in the center. Provide a table behind the leader to hold supplies. A swivel chair with wheels will help the facilitator to navigate through the group while staying at residents' eye level.

As a facilitator, you should begin the group in the same manner every week. Welcome each member individually and tell him or her your name at each introduction. Tell each resident that you are glad he or she is here and glad that he or she is part of the Connections group. Make sure each resident is seated in the same location every week.

Begin by handing an item to each participant, taking time with the item and the resident. Do not identify the item, but discuss the item with the resident. Ask him or her about the use and purpose of the item. It does not matter if the resident identifies the item correctly. If he or she does, congratulate and praise without going overboard. Leave the item with the resident and proceed to the next resident with the next item. Continue this process, until all the residents have an item with which to work. Encourage them to help each other to identify the items. Promote working as a team and finding the answers together. Once the residents have identified their items separately, ask them for a single word that describes all these items. The single word that sums up the "connection" is not as important as the group involvement, discussion and participation leading up to that word. Praise the participants often.

Make sure the group *does not* insult a resident's intelligence. I have not had many residents feel insulted or hurt by this group. Most of their reactions have been positive. The facilitator will know immediately if this group is inappropriate for a new resident. This group can be used as an evaluation tool. Invite new residents in for a session. If it is obvious that the group is inappropriate for a resident, encourage that person to help the others. This way, he or she can feel a sense of pride, and maybe start a friendship during that initial visit. You can place the resident more appropriately next time, and they haven't wasted their first session with you. Many better-oriented residents enjoy this group because the interaction involved is valuable to them despite the simplicity of the group. Store the items in plastic containers and stack the boxes in your supply cabinet. Clearly identify each "connection" box. These boxes can also be used as part of a room visit.

> *Katie was a classy dresser. We placed her in Connections on her second day at the facility. She was very verbal and was able to identify almost all the items that were presented to her. She identified the items with pride and was able to help the other residents with clues and words to augment what the facilitator was saying. Katie also had a beautiful voice and sang "Memories" at the end of the group the first day. Needless to say we continued to invite Katie to the group and she began and ended every group with this song. She went as far as to teach the other members the song. She was probably "too oriented" for the group, but she loved it. This was her place to be successful.*

Chapter Four

Trivia Time

Trivia Time provides an opportunity for cognitively impaired residents to respond to simple trivia questions. The group allows members to answer questions created for their level of ability, and is designed mainly for reality orientation. Day, time and place must be discussed at every meeting. Keeping residents focused on the group's goal is important to the stability of the group.

Goal: To provide trivia as entertainment, and as a tool to stimulate communication and simple discussion.

Objectives:

- Tailor every question to the abilities of the group;

- Provide the opportunity to talk and be listened to, no matter what the topic;

- Reinforce time, date and season during every group (reality orientation);

- Offer an opportunity to use long-term and short-term memory;

- Provide an avenue for the resident with an interest in events and trivia; and

- Concentrate and listen to full sentences and a few directions.

Group Content and Setup

Trivia is only the catalyst to make this group work. Examples of trivia will not be provided in this book, since there are so many sources from which to draw. The trivia must be very simple, and should be related to the interests of the participants. Assessment of each resident and their interests is very important for the success of Trivia Time.

Section 1—Introduction (3–5 minutes)
Residents are asked the same questions at the beginning of every group:

- "What is the day?"

- "What is the year?"

- "What is the season?" and

- "What is the weather like outside today?"

This provides reality orientation for the group. If reality orientation is a goal for a specific resident, Trivia Time would be an acceptable intervention. If you can, use a chalkboard to write out each question. Writing the residents' answers on the board empowers them to become more involved and take more ownership of the group. It is excellent, too, if one of the residents can write the answers on the board, but that is not always possible.

Section 2—Get Acquainted (10–12 minutes)
Next, help residents get acquainted with each other and ask the following questions:

- "Who is beside you?"

- "Who is across from you?"

- "How many people named Mary are in the group?"

- "How many people are in the group?"

- "What day comes after Friday?" or

- "What season comes after winter?"

These questions can usually be repeated, and directed individually to more than one participant without the residents getting bored.

Section 3—Trivia (10–15 minutes)
This begins the simple trivia portion of the group. Seasonal, thematic, presidential or other trivia can be used in this section.

Ideally, this group is seated classroom style. The number of participants in this group can be as high as ten. Trivia Time works best when participants have similar interests. A blackboard or a marker board should be used to display questions first, then the answers to the questions. The board is easier to read if everyone is facing it. Prepare the questions in advance with all of them written out in your notes.

The group should last 30 minutes. This is a success-oriented group. Prizes and competition might even be introduced if the group becomes popular. Assess the residents accurately and make sure you match the demands of participation carefully with each resident's abilities. Be careful not to invite someone who is too advanced for the group. *Do not* make the questions too difficult. This group can be a lot of fun for residents if it is run properly. You may want to try a version of Trivia Time for higher functioning residents as well, so you might also classify this as an interest-based group.

Radio Daze and Movie Mania

These two groups use popular media from days gone by as a catalyst. The groups are designed to help residents with limited recall and limited long-term memories reminisce about radio shows and movies. Each is very structured.

Goal: To increase memory recall, recognition and attention span.

Objectives:

- The opportunity to focus and center in on one issue;
- Hear old, familiar shows;
- Increase use of long-term and short-term memory skills; and
- Socialize and share stories about radio broadcasts and movies.

Select residents for these groups who enjoy old movies or radio shows. Group members should have adequate hearing, since the audiotapes and videotapes are more enjoyable if one can clearly hear what is going on. The timing of the group is crucial for the residents with a short attention span. Keep the group moving and allow for the group to direct where it wants to go.

Group Content and Setup

The consistent format for Radio Daze and Movie Mania is the key to the residents' success. The groups should be run in exactly the same fashion every week except for the program content selected for the entertainment portion of the meeting. The group begins with one member handing out nametags to the group. The facilitator can have the nametags ready and escort the "helper" around the room, aiding in identification of the group members. Everyone wears a nametag.

Radio Daze/Movie Mania Agenda:

1. Welcome and nametags
2. Pictures
3. Radio or movie segment
4. Discussion
5. Questions
6. Conclusion and summary

Chapter Four

The facilitator begins by passing around pictures of old radios, movie projectors, and pictures of celebrities and personalities that the residents are familiar with, which sets the tone in a fun and friendly manner. Encourage discussion of the pictures and residents' memories of what is depicted in the pictures. The residents do not usually get bored, as long as the pictures change from time to time. The pictures should be laminated and be able to be passed easily from resident to resident. Stick to one theme, time period, or specific show to help continuity.

After viewing and discussing the pictures, the group listens to a radio show or watches a small part of a famous movie. There are quite a few sources for audiotapes and videotapes. Your public library may be the best of all. This portion of the group will last approximately fifteen minutes. Discussion follows, centered on the program you have presented. It is important to keep the conversation directed, but allow residents to discuss whatever part of the show they would like. Encourage members to listen to one another as much as to talk. Repeat key words from a resident's statements, so all can understand the conversation better. Group conversation seems to be improved if the facilitator stands or walks among the group members and stimulates conversation with simple questions when it starts to lag.

When conversation dies down, the facilitator can keep things moving by asking questions. Make them simple and have them relate directly to the fifteen minutes of the show you listened to or movie you watched. A very popular movie in this setting is *The Wizard of Oz*. The first fifteen minutes of this movie is in black and white. Play the movie until the color comes on. There are plenty of trivia questions the facilitator can ask about the show such as, "Where did Dorothy go when she ran away?" If the residents participating in these groups have different levels of abilities, you can prepare a variety of simple to difficult questions prior to the group. At the end of the questions, everyone is thanked for coming and reminded of next week's meeting.

Do not offer Radio Daze and Movie Mania simultaneously. You should begin with one and stick with it for three to six months. When you are getting started, offering Movie Mania is easier. It is often difficult for residents to just sit and listen. Sometimes they need to relearn how to listen without any visual stimulus.

Just as with Trivia Time, you should be flexible with Radio Daze and Movie Mania, and be prepared to schedule sessions of these groups for higher functioning residents as an interest-based group. We have had many residents interested in this group because of their personal interest in movies. Often, residents will want to watch or listen for more than fifteen minutes. That should be anticipated. Make sure all affected departments know that these group meetings might run over their scheduled time, but don't allow the group to run for more than 90 minutes.

It helps if your facilitator has some interest in old movies or radio shows. It makes it more interesting for the residents if the facilitator can answer questions they might have. This group can be the most enjoyable one to lead.

Chapter Four

The Work Group

Dick, a retired construction worker, lived in the Alzheimer's unit at our facility. Dick was always walking around and working on various and sundry areas. Usually he had an imaginary tool and was digging at the wall or floor. It was extremely difficult to redirect him. When we thought about placing Dick in The Work Group, we were unsure as to his abilities. We tried many different diversions with him, and for the longest time nothing seemed to get him distracted enough to stop his tearing wallpaper off the wall or pushing up the carpet. Then one day, I was cleaning a table after an activity and Dick came up to me. He seemed to be watching every move I made. I was using Windex on the tables, hoping to remove a stain. I knew I couldn't let Dick use the spray bottle I was using, so I found an empty spray bottle and put water in it. I gave him a roll of paper towels and the water spray bottle and asked him to help me with the tables. He caught on immediately and began wiping down the tables. He was instinctively excellent at this job. He didn't need any coaching, or any help. He was able to feel extremely needed and purposeful every breakfast, lunch and dinner following that day. He truly excelled, and he knew at last he was doing something useful again.

The Work Group provides an outlet for residents with cognitive impairments who need direction and work-oriented projects. Opportunities to feel useful and productive help the resident. Select residents who like to stay busy, perhaps those who wander the halls or those who seem to have some excess energy. Assessments help to select the residents who have enjoyed working all their life and find fulfillment in "keeping busy." There are homemakers, as well as workaholics, that will participate in any activity just to stay busy.

Goals: To provide an environment that contributes and fulfills the residents' need to work and provides a sense of purpose to their lives.

Objectives:

- Help residents who have a difficult time being idle;

- Provide normalcy and relevance in the lives of participants;

- Increase participants' independence and self-esteem; and

- Provide satisfying jobs to residents who are willing and eager to work.

The Work Group is usually a very small group. All of its members have a history of work and community involvement. They are physically active residents. Our goal is to create a failure-free group. The main focus of The Work Group is what interests the resident—what they did before they retired; the hobbies they have enjoyed. For membership in The Work Group to be a positive experience, it is important that the resident can be taught routine tasks. Helping with distribution of magazines or snacks, for instance, can make a resident feel very useful. Once members are properly directed, often they can perform independently. For those who need support, help or encouragement, the weekly meeting should include the facilitator. Keeping three or four residents involved in the same work group allows for diversity, companionship and socialization.

Group Content and Setup

The tasks assigned to members might change as their skills and ability levels change. Offering simple instruction, patience and kindness will make The Work Group succeed. Many of the tasks assigned to members will need coordination with other departments. Make sure you take everyone's needs into account, so you provide a positive situation for the resident and the people involved in helping out. Explain the needs and abilities of the resident to the staff you will be recruiting. Housekeeping and maintenance can help fulfill the needs of the work-oriented resident. They must understand why you are involving them and their department.

The following is a list of the work groups and tasks we have used:

- Magazine carts
- Dusting
- Food carts
- Folding bibs

- Sweeping inside and outside the facility
- Emptying waste cans
- Preparing morning coffee

37

- Cleaning handrails
- Cleaning tables
- Cleaning windows
- Washing and drying plastic cups and dishes
- Polishing shoes
- Folding shirt protectors
- Folding towels
- Washing chairs
- Helping transport residents to activities or the beauty parlor
- Delivering mail

- Setting tables
- Cleaning bingo/poker chips
- Stuffing envelopes
- Decorating bulletin boards
- Delivering papers
- Raking
- Weeding
- Watering flowers inside and outside the facility
- Passing out coffee or cookies (with gloves on)
- Moving a square on a large facility calendar each day

Food carts probably need some explanation. This can be an innovative and involving group activity. A cart on wheels is the mode of transportation for special food to the resident. Most activity services departments have access to a cart. Each person is assigned an area in which he or she delivers food from room to room.

I like to offer a food cart to all residents once a week. It can be recorded as a room visit or a therapeutic group, depending on the situation. Food carts are coordinated by activity services with advice from the food services department and the dietician.

Themes tend to be successful. They are also a helpful way to think of a food item for the cart. Themes are so often related to food, as you can see in these examples:

- Thanksgiving—Pumpkin pie
- Christmas—Christmas pudding, fruit cake
- Summér—Strawberry shortcake, peach pie
- Oktoberfest—German chocolate cake, dill pickles
- Orange Days (color days)—Oranges (a theme-colored food)

- International Chocolate Chip Cookie Day

- Brownie Day

- Coca-Cola Day

Some things to keep in mind are:

- Have alternatives for all dietary needs.

- When scheduling the food cart, allow plenty of time for delivery of service.

This is a great opportunity to involve one of your Work Group members to help deliver the cart from room to room. He or she is able to prepare the items outside the room and stay with the cart when your staff goes into the room with the food. It is enjoyable for your helpers to feel useful, and they really do make the job easier.

The Work Group can prove to be the most time-consuming group developed. It involves just a few of the more capable residents, but the projects are lengthy at times and it's nearly impossible to leave a resident alone to complete the task. You are looking at the equivalent of a very long room visit—out of their room. The fulfillment the resident experiences far outweighs the potential problems and the staff time devoted to the group and its members. Using other personnel in the facility and community volunteers or family members can take some of the load off an activity services staff with time constraints.

Light Touch

Light Touch is a simple massage group. Participants meet once a week for personal one-on-one attention. The group provides soothing music and a comfortable environment in which to relax. Participants experience the act of touching and relaxation. Only involve residents who like to be touched, and give preference to those who have little contact with family or friends. Residents who do not like to be touched are easily identified and should *not* be included in this group. Touching should *never* occur without the permission or invitation of the resident.

Goals: To provide an opportunity for intimacy through music and touch on an unconditional basis.

Objectives:

- Provide one-on-one attention in a group setting;

- Provide touch where not much touch is experienced;

- Promote relaxation; and

- Provide intimacy.

Touch is not something that all people like. It is very important to make sure your group members will enjoy participating. You may need to involve the resident's family to tell you more about the resident's past lifestyle. Touch is one thing that is sadly lacking from the nursing home resident's daily routine. Light Touch is a very simple therapeutic group that has great benefits.

Group Content and Setup

Begin and end the group with classical music or "environmental sound" tapes that are widely available. The music or background tape can continue throughout the entire session. Once you have found music that the group enjoys, use the same music for several weeks in a row. The group should be in a circle and should not involve more than four or five residents. The group members should be placed very close to each other.

Prepare warm, wet washcloths (heat six in the microwave for one minute) and wash the hands of all the group members. Even if a resident can wash his or her own hands, offer to help. Complementing the fact that he or she can wash his or her own hands will help to promote independence. This group should never decrease independence of a resident in any way. Supply one bottle of hand lotion for each resident, marked with his or her name. Use the lotion to rub the hands of each resident.

The length of time you spend with each resident is up to you. After both hands have been cleaned and rubbed with lotion, ask the group members to follow a few simple directions. See if they can rub their hands together. Ask them to lift their hands, separate their fingers, stretch their fingers. Keep it simple, and do not massage more than the hands. See Sit and Be Fit in chapter six for further hand-massage techniques (page 110).

Have residents who are unable to participate in other groups be a part of this group. Do not worry if there doesn't seem to be a lot happening in the group. Let the residents relax, and enjoy being part of this quiet group.

Chapter Four

Name Game

The Name Game provides the opportunity for residents to identify their name, to become aware of their environment, and to learn the names of the other residents in the group.

Goal: To establish an opportunity to help identify the resident's name and the names of other group members.

Objectives:

- See their own name in print and learn to identify it;

- Promote saying their own name;

- Help recognize written letters, their name and the names of other residents in the group; and

- Establish a social situation that allows participants to help one another.

Jewell was a woman who spoke only angry words. The staff felt that she had led a very sad and lonely life. She was placed in the Name Game because she had very low cognitive functioning. More than that, though, we just didn't know where else to put her. She acted inappropriately, and sometimes even aggressively in group settings.

She was immediately able to identify her own name. She was also able to identify the names of the rest of the group members. One day, as she sat waiting for lunch to be served, she leaned over and said to her tablemate and fellow group member, "Lucy, can you say your name?" Jewell had finally come out of her shell. Over time, Jewell began handing out the nametags to each of the group members. She began teaching the other members of the group how to say their names and how to read their names. Now that she had learned to work appropriately in a group, she was able to move on. Name Game and the vulnerability of its members had allowed her to develop social skills without feeling threatened.

Group Content and Setup

The facilitator needs to prepare for this group by using a computer or typewriter, and a copier. The first and last names of the residents should be typed or printed from a word-processing program, and cleanly photocopied in several sizes. Create four or five examples of each name in sizes varying from one-inch to eight-inches high. Make sure you use the same font for each name. Avoid italics since they are more difficult to read. It is advisable to laminate all the nametags. Make sure the facilitator has a nametag for himself or herself, too. All the names are placed in a basket that is used solely for this group. The names of the residents are also put on a single, large piece of paper.

No more than five or six residents participate in this group. The group can be in a circle, but a table is helpful so that names can be placed in front of each member. The group lasts one half-hour and should begin with introductions and a welcome by the facilitator.

We also begin and end with the song "The More We Get Together" (sung to the tune of "Have You Ever Seen a Lassie") using the names of the group members:

> *The more we get together, together, together,*
> *The more we get together, the happier we will be.*
> *There is Mary.... and John.... and Sue....*
> *The more we get together the happier we will be.*
> *There is Robert.... and Tina.... and Jewell....*
> *Happy, happy, happy we will be.*

This reinforces their names and puts music into the group. To start a session, the facilitator will present the names individually to each resident. Slowly the facilitator will hold up the name so it is visible to the group (using the largest copy first) and ask the resident to hold up his or her name. It can be a very slow process. The first task is to identify that it is his or her name. It is helpful to have the resident hold the large print name and see if he or she can tell you what it says. If that is possible for the resident, use the next smaller size, to determine the extent of his or her visual capabilities.

If the resident can identify his or her own name, ask him or her to identify the other members of the group. Using the full group list of names, see if he or she can read all the names of the group members. After you read the name of a group member, ask the participants to point to that person. Also make sure that they can identify the facilitator. Continue this process and see if each group member can begin to identify his or her own name and the names of others.

43

Chapter Four

Make sure the residents in this group are very low functioning. If they are able to identify their name and the names of the members of the group easily, then the next step would be to place them in another therapeutic group such as Connections. An alternative to this group process is to use these names prior to lunch or dinner with the residents coming into the room and preparing for a meal.

Fred was a wanderer. He was only calm when his wife came to visit but since he was almost uncontrollable when she left, she visited irregularly. Fred was hard to direct, and was seldom interested in anything. He enjoyed punchball, but after a few minutes he would become bored and restless. He would just get up and leave. One day we were playing Name Game. Fred came and stood beside me. I handed him the name of a resident and immediately he called out the name, "Anna Smith." Everyone in the room turned around and immediately quieted down and listened to him.

He didn't shout or yell, Fred just commanded attention. He had the entire dining room in the palm of his hand. He was so happy and overwhelmed with the response. He went up to Anna Smith and said, "I am glad you recognized your name, and I hope you can put this name somewhere in your house so you can enjoy it." Fred continued to hand out the names and discussed each name with each resident. This was a great way to keep the group busy while the other staff brought the residents in for lunch and it seemed to relax the residents to hold their names in their hands. Fred ended up doing this every lunch time and felt like he had a job every day. He always showed up for work.

Spell and Tell

Spell and Tell has been very successful for many reasons. The residents involved only have to identify letters and words. This is a learned process and much like riding a bike. It is often a skill we retain despite other losses experienced as we age. This spelling group is multileveled and appeals to many people. It is a good icebreaker. It is a wonderful tool to attract the retired teachers, businessmen and homemakers who are familiar with the props used.

Goal: To provide an opportunity for residents with visual impairments or low cognitive ability to spell words and rekindle their interest in words and the alphabet.

Objectives:

- Provoke long-term memory with letters, words and names;

- Identify letters and short words;

- Spell or correct inaccurate spelling of words;

- Spell their first and last name; and

- Spell the name of the items presented.

Group Content and Setup

The only prop needed for this small group is a set of magnetic boards. This will allow the participants to have their own board and to spell the words they are asked to spell. The magnetic board must have colorful magnetic letters (more than just 26) included with the board.

The difficulty level of these tasks presents a starting point and a set of goals for participants. Spell and Tell works well as an assessment tool. It can help you place residents in groups that are appropriate for their cognitive levels. The more they are able to do on the hierarchy of objectives, the more they will be able to participate in a higher cognitive group like Trivia Time. This is a set of simple tasks. These tasks tend to separate the residents who can comprehend simple directions and have long-term memory from those who do not.

The residents find the magnetic boards easier to use if they are sitting around a table. This limits the number in the group to four to six. It is easy to facilitate by simply walking around the table as you call out a word. Start with three-letter words. Don't be disappointed if you don't ever get any farther. Make sure the words you use are familiar, such as:

ape	bun	cat	dog
egg	far	got	keg
hat	lab	man	nut
pen	rib	sit	ten
van	win	zoo	

or simply place an item, such as a cup on the table and see if they can identify and spell. Then add to the difficulty by adding a letter. For example, pose this question to the group: What letter can you add to 'pen' to make another word?" Have the vowels in front of them—try each vowel. They will undoubtedly come up with the correct answer. Common four- or five-letter words can also be successful, but the group will let you know when and if it is too difficult.

Make sure part of each group involves participants spelling their own first and last names. One group session can simply be family names. This has proven to be successful.

The amazing part of this therapeutic group is the response it can evoke from previously unresponsive residents. Participation here can be determined by a resident's success in the Name Game group. In that group setting, the main objective is to identify one's own written and spoken name. This just goes one step further and rekindles the knowledge of letters and words with sometimes surprising results. Spell and Tell has a simple structure and not much variety. The half-hour goes by in a hurry.

> *Ruth is an 80-year-old resident with dementia, described by all as jovial and friendly. She responds phenomenally to music and can be quite lucid in one-on-one conversation. In her first session of Spell and Tell, she was asked to spell the word BED. She simply could not do it. She could identify the word, but just could not spell it. This word and a few other similar three-letter words were presented to her for a period of weeks, without much result. On the sixth week she was asked to spell the word DOG, which she had not worked with prior to this meeting. She picked up the letters and spelled DOG correctly. She proceeded in the following weeks to spell all the three-letter words correctly. She had relearned the concept of spelling and she performed wonderfully. She could never spell words longer than three letters, but she felt successful and proud. So were we.*

You might be surprised, as I was, to hear from staff that quite a few residents not invited to the group wanted to take part in Spell and Tell. The higher cognitive resident is very interested in using the board in a different way. He or she will use the board to answer questions such as, "What kind of day is it today?" This is a form of reality orientation, but residents are not aware that they are being questioned, and seem not to feel "cornered." The oriented resident finds it interesting to spell his or her own name and the name of the facility. The activity services staff can initiate a relationship between a resident who is oriented and the less-oriented residents, by asking them to help. Simple questions can be asked and the oriented resident can explain the answers to the other residents.

High-Functioning Groups  5

I was surprised, and a little puzzled. I had never seen Dan show much emotion, but there he was, tears streaming down his face. And it didn't seem like any time to be crying. We were on an outing. A bus full of residents was going to "Day at the Races" at a nearby horse track. I leaned over to Dan and whispered, "Are you all right?" Dan looked up and simply said, "I never thought I'd be able to do anything like this again. Thank you."

Groups discussed in this chapter—

- One-On-One

- Storylines

- Reflections

- Memory Lane—or "Where Is Your Neighborhood?"

- Today's News

- Faith, Hope and Charity

- Pen Pals

- Hospitality Club

- A Special Friend—An Intergenerational Connection

- Spelling Bee

You have to consider that life in a nursing home can be pretty boring. For a resident with no significant mental limitations, it can get downright depressing. There is often a complete lack of challenge for someone who is oriented, able and aware. These residents see everything that is happening around them, but due to their physical limitations they are not considered "normal" to our society. Often their opinions and advice are not taken seriously, because they live in a nursing home and "could not possibly have vital, important opinions." The more activity services staff can do to provide a normal living environment for each individual, the closer we are to offering the best possible quality of life. Normalization is a major goal for the activity professional's work with the oriented resident.

Being aware and alert might just be the most difficult personal situation for a nursing home resident. Being aware is not always a blessing when a resident is dealing with a disease that slowly takes away their ability to function independently.

I spent a lot of time with a retired engineer named Arthur when I was working in Florida. Arthur made me think about groups for the high-functioning resident. We had many discussions about his work and his life. He was a valued member of his community, and was involved in designing and building a large portion of Interstate 75. He was very educated, and yet very lonely. As Arthur received treatment for his incurable cancer, we often discussed which was worse—being mentally limited or physically limited. It was important to Arthur to have a purpose, to have a reason for living, and to be needed by someone.

Arthur's wife had died five years earlier. He had few family visitors. He needed a job. A work group wouldn't be fulfilling to him. He needed a real *job. His one true love was to share his memories and experiences working on those huge highway projects. I began introducing him to other residents, some not as talkative as Arthur, but equally work-oriented. He established some meaningful relationships. This was the beginning of my first therapeutic group for oriented and involved residents. The peer group called One-On-One was born.*

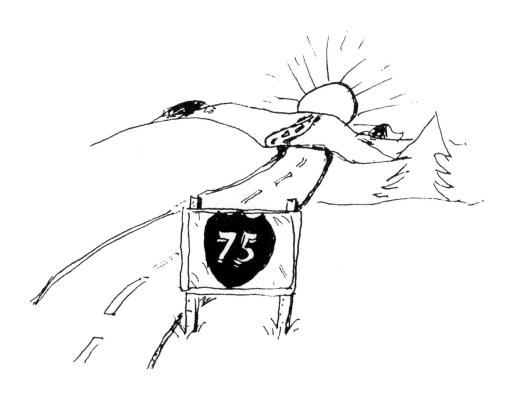

One-On-One

Goal: To establish a relationship between two residents—an oriented resident (visitor) and a resident who is room-bound or in need of visitors and friends (host).

Objectives:

- Provide the visitor an opportunity to help in the facility;

- Allow visitors to meet on a regular basis and discuss someone other than themselves;

- Encourage development of leadership skills;

- Provide an opportunity to discuss personal issues in a non-threatening environment; and

- Provide social interaction for the host.

Group Content and Setup

This therapeutic group is structured around the group of oriented residents (visitors) who meet weekly to discuss their visits with room-bound residents (hosts). The social service department should be involved to oversee the group or serve as speakers for the group. The topics that are covered in the weekly meeting vary greatly from week to week. The group facilitator provides a selection of topics, but usually group members channel the discussion where they want it to go. The following are suggested topics for the regular meeting. The meeting lasts no longer than 30 minutes. This time restriction is important since these residents like to organize their day. Stick with the same day, facilitator, time and length of group and you are sure to have regular attendance and participation. The facilitator will know if the group is ready for these topics, or whether they need more instruction on how to conduct their visits:

- What does it mean to be a visitor?

- What responsibilities are involved?

- What am I supposed to do and not do?

This is a good opportunity to discuss what should happen during a visit. The first visit to each room-bound resident should involve a social service or activity services staff member. This will allow the visitor to ask questions and ask for recommendations if the visit does not go as planned. The responsibilities of the visitor should be discussed at every meeting. It is important for the visitor to understand that his or her visit could be the only one that the host is receiving. That helps the visitors appreciate the importance of the role they have agreed to take on.

- How do you visit someone?

- What do you actually do during a room visit?

- What have you done that has been successful? That was not successful?

Each "veteran" in the group needs to discuss what he or she has experienced and obstacles he or she has encountered. Visitors may encounter comments such as:

- I am in pain, what should I do?

- I would just like to die.

- Why is my family not visiting me?

- I wish my roommate would quit...

These are difficult topics and need to be dealt with individually and openly. Use every issue brought up by your visitors as a new discussion topic. Each new topic can be brought to the social service department. Your social service department should do research for a presentation at a future meeting.

Choose one of the group members to share a story every week. Ask him or her well in advance of the meeting and he or she will feel more comfortable giving the presentation. Given a chance to prepare, he or she will be eager to share their experience. This helps other group members to open up about what has happened as they visited. The facilitator should be prepared to lead role-playing to help visitors prepare for what they might encounter if the stories do not stimulate sufficient discussion with the group members.

Social service personnel should be involved in this exercise from the beginning. Do not wait until situations develop. Social service staff can help focus on the group members' accomplishments, and help them avoid getting discouraged by the illnesses and the problems they encounter. Activity services staff must be dedicated to keeping the group interested in each other and their visits. Try to provide daily encouragement, reminders and ideas whenever you encounter one of your visitors.

Chapter Five

One-On-One can help your facility meet state requirements for room visits to room-bound residents. Effective documentation is important to achieving this extra benefit. Provide calendars for the activity services staff to monitor participation of visitors and hosts, just as you would for other volunteers. A copy of a simple one-page monthly calendar can be placed in both the visitor's and the host's charts. This allows you to document increased socialization for a room-bound resident or maintenance of leadership skills for the visitor. Your care plan for each visitor should list the number of visits he or she will do weekly.

Visitors should be given responsibility for their own calendars. Calendars should be handed out at the first meeting each month. This provides a perfect opportunity for discussion on how visits are going and problems that might be occurring. Each calendar is clearly marked with the name of the resident being visited, for example: "Duane's Visiting Schedule." Each time a visit occurs, the visitor signs his or her name. (See Appendix A for sample calendar.) The calendar can be a visual cue, something for the host to hang on his or her bulletin board as a reminder of his or her schedule. This calendar is also valuable as a reminder to the hosts of other visits from the community and from their family. This helps them recall all the visits of the month. If the host is lonely and states "no one is visiting me," the activity services staff can show the host his or her calendar and review the visits together.

One-On-One lets you get maximum use of your resources. You are providing benefit for each host by way of weekly or biweekly visits. You are also helping each of your visitors to *be* independent and *stay* independent. With a group membership of six, and with each member visiting two residents per week, you are helping 18 of your residents, with a regular commitment to just one group meeting a week.

One-On-One can be a big commitment for the visitor. The group's facilitator must monitor relationships. There is a twofold purpose to watching over these relationships as they develop. It helps the visitor keep a healthy perspective. It also helps room-bound residents to develop realistic expectations. Each new relationship should be supervised at first. Once visits are held without supervision, the facilitator should talk privately with the visitor. Sometimes, visitors need to talk about their experiences immediately following a visit, rather than waiting for the weekly One-On-One meeting. Confidentiality has not proven to be a problem, as the visitors do not share the name of their host, just the situation. Only the facilitator and the visitor know of whom they are speaking. When this group is working well, important relationships will be created. I have seen a simple visit, a weekly reading of the Bible to a blind resident, become a deep and committed personal relationship. One-On-One can make a big difference to everyone involved.

Summary of One-On-One

1. Visitors are assigned one or two host(s) and one or two visits per week.

2. Visitors are responsible for hosts' calendars handed out at the first meeting every month. This calendar can be used in both residents' charts (host for room visit documentation; visitor for leadership/facility involvement documentation).

3. Visits should last no longer than 15 minutes. Visits can begin with two or three simple, short introductory meetings accompanied by the group facilitator.

4. Limit hosts to only one visitor/host relationship at a time because host could show favoritism and hurt visitor's feelings.

5. Facilitator is responsible for keeping enthusiasm high for visitors by reinforcing their importance and praising their success' throughout the week.

Storylines

Sometimes, life is not a laughing matter. Then again, sometimes it is. Our Storylines group had been meeting for over a year. People came and went, but the core group remained the same. They had presented a Thanksgiving prayer and a Christmas poem to the rest of the facility. The group had their own costumes. Through all this, they had become personally very close. The winter months brought bad news, however. With ten active members, five passed away within two months. This devastated the group. The facilitator understood the group dynamics, and spent two months with the group in mourning. The group went to the funerals together, prayed together, and shared great stories about the lost members. This was the most powerful way to deal with death I have ever seen. If only every resident could be remembered as these people remembered their friends. This difficult time brought out the true value of Storylines to its members.

Goal: To provide a stimulating, challenging, interpersonal situation for the resident.

Objectives:

- Provide challenges not offered to residents in their day-to-day life;

- Help increase mental capabilities;

- Provide opportunities to use the imagination;

- Improve memory skills;

- Promote relationships in the group;

- Provide opportunities to make choices and judgments about important personal issues; and

- Promote socialization.

Group Content and Setup

Storylines is designed to challenge members' minds and generate interest, involvement and creative thought. The group meets weekly and has as many as ten members, all alert and oriented, possibly with diverse backgrounds and interests. The group usually lasts 30 minutes, but during play practice more time may be needed. They must share a need to be social and to be challenged. Residents involved in diversionary groups such as bingo and game time often participate in Storylines. This group adds a new dimension to life in the nursing home.

Make sure the following jobs are filled each week:

- **Greeter:** This member is the first person group members see upon their arrival. The Greeter welcomes the group and tells them the date, time and location of the meeting.

- **Nametag Writer:** This member needs appropriate supplies, and prepares nametags for each member at each meeting.

- **Secretary/Reviewer of Past Events:** This member holds the position for an entire month. He or she records news and happenings of the group and reports what "homework" should be turned in at this meeting. (Homework is described later in this section.)

- **Introducer:** This member introduces all the other members by first and last name—this develops memory skills.

- **Summarizer:** At the conclusion of each meeting, this member thanks everyone for coming and summarizes the events that have occurred during the group.

- **Homework Man:** Hands out the homework the facilitator and/or group has prepared every week.

What must be understood is that the "jobs" listed above are handed out with humor and fun. The facilitator must often take a job temporarily, and instruct the members on its simplicity. The jobs (except the Secretary) may be rotated on a weekly basis. The shyest members can begin with the easier jobs.

The program is simple and it can be adjusted to meet the needs of the group. Many memory games can be played:

- Place items in a bag and ask the group to identify them by feeling the items in the bag without seeing them.

- Place items on a tray. Hide the tray, remove one item and ask the group which item is removed.

- Place an item on the table. Ask each resident to talk about the item for one minute.

- Give an obscure word to a resident. Ask him or her to invent a definition, or come up with the real definition, and convince the group of its correctness.

- Ask questions about the roles within in the group: "Who was the greeter last week; who was the homework man two weeks ago?"

Homework is key to this group. The process begins very simply by asking each member to remember a word or short phrase until the next meeting. You might begin by asking the member their favorite color and adding a noun: for example, red convertible. Step up the complexity of the homework a little bit each week. When one of the members is ill, it is the responsibility of the group to meet with the absent member, tell him or her their homework and review the group's meeting for him or her.

Important components to remember each week:

1. Nametags are a must—and a very important part of this process. Tags must be prepared each week in the same format as the group members arrive.

2. Facilitate only—do not lead.

3. Hold meetings in the same location, on the same day, and at the same time each week.

4. Give members the responsibility to get to the group on their own accord.

5. Homework will be handed out every week.

6. Give duties to all members as assignments rotate. Responsibility helps increase self-esteem.

7. Change the duties periodically, and let members assign jobs when and as they wish. A poster or erasable marker board listing the job titles is helpful when it is time to rotate assignments.

The memory games played during each meeting form the foundation for word memory projects. Those projects will be central to the group's purpose. I have had remarkable success with this group memorizing famous poetry. After weeks of practice, Storylines presented a well-known poem as a group in front of the entire nursing home. Beyond that, you might try a play, a humorous short story or historical reenactment. Go slowly, because there is no rush to reach any particular goal. Your residents will tell you how much they are willing to do.

Some objectives for goal setting and care planning for this group are:

- Learn to listen and repeat homework on a weekly basis;

- Remember a certain number of words or phrases weekly;

- Get to know the other residents in a more constructive way;

- Help each other increase their self-awareness and their sensory awareness;

- Test and help increase their memory potential;

- Be aware of their surroundings;

- Feel useful by performing a job within the group;

- Develop their sense of imagination;

- Learn to interact with one another;

- Learn to trust; and

- Prepare and present a skit or a presentation once a year.

Reflections: A Reminiscing Group

Reflections is designed to provide a social situation promoting discussion and friendship. Facilitators will provide multimedia props to help the group recall meaningful moments in their lives.

Goal: To provide an opportunity for members to recall their past with participants of similar age and attitude.

Objectives:

- Use past experiences to utilize long-term memory;

- Bring memories into their lives and allow those memories to be accepted and praised;

- Provide closure for issues that have not been satisfactorily resolved; and

- Provide an opportunity to think of happy thoughts and good memories and share them with a group.

Group Content and Setup

When properly managed, Reflections is an energizing experience for residents. The use of memory aids like music, old magazines, newspapers, and tapes of radio shows can be a major memory booster. Keep in mind that *discussion* is the reason for the group, and don't let the props take over.

Many reminiscing groups are currently offered in long-term care and open to all residents. It is best to invite specific residents to this group. Group members will end up taking ownership of the group. Keep participation requirements firmly in mind when issuing invitations. If residents that really don't belong are invited, it can cause people to "shut down," and even become angry if the flow of conversation is interrupted by inappropriate behavior.

Set the ground rules when the group begins and review them at the beginning of every meeting. Have the group decide on the rules and post them during meetings.

Rules that work well:

- There are no limits on discussion topics;

- Everyone gets the opportunity to speak;

- Allow the other person in the group to finish speaking;

- Do not correct people for inaccuracies;

- Do not take over the group—no one speaks for more than two minutes;

- What is discussed in the group, stays in the group.

The concept for Reflections is already used quite widely in the nursing home environment. Unfortunately, the concept is often poorly applied. Do not strive for variety in the group's membership. High-functioning residents can become resentful if the flow of the group is disrupted by lower functioning residents. Keep each meeting to a single theme, such as family life, movies, sports, politics, music. Topics must be planned in advance, and props located. Future topics should be discussed at the end of each group. The residents should decide on the next week's topic and can be delegated to handle part of the presentation.

It is a good idea to invite a social service representative to be part of this group. This activity is closest to a group therapy concept discussed in this book (see chapter eight for more information on group therapy in a nursing home). Emotions and memories can be brought forward that activity services staff are not trained or prepared to handle. The group can be a useful outlet for the residents who have issues to discuss. For the most part it's good fun, but expect some surprises.

Some topics that work well:

- Prices of items in the 1930s;

- Occupations;

- Transportation and how it has changed;

- Raising a family;

- Household appliances; and

- The pros and cons of travelling.

Chapter Five

Memory Lane—Or "Where Is Your Neighborhood?"

Group transportation, such as a van or a bus, is a vital component of any successful activity program. Transportation allows residents to experience the community. Any activity program can be more beneficial when group transportation is available. Taking residents out into the community is a marvelous way to enhance normalization. You make a substantial improvement in quality of life when you help your residents to experience reality beyond the walls of the nursing home.

Memory Lane is designed for the oriented nursing home resident who still lives in his or her hometown. It only works for the resident who is able to verbalize and has long-term and short-term memory. As you can guess from the group's name, Memory Lane involves driving residents through the areas where they used to live, go to school, shop and enjoy themselves. For maximum benefit, trips should be thoroughly planned, based on information you gather from your residents.

Goal: To provide the opportunity for normalization and integration in the community in a normal and comfortable setting. To provide the fulfillment of seeing a place the residents called home or are familiar with.

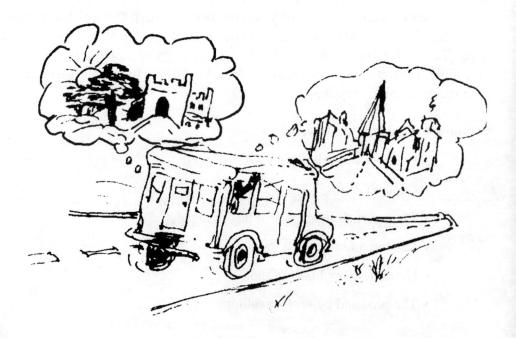

Objectives:

- Provide transportation to local areas of interest;

- Provide interesting trips around the area;

- Offer the opportunity to rekindle places of the past;

- Allow the residents to feel good about where they lived and spent time; and

- Use memory skills to share memories with other residents.

Group Content and Setup

By asking a few pertinent questions during your initial assessment you can identify your high-cognitive residents without much trouble, and do the research you need to plan your Memory Lane trips. There is some preliminary work to do before the trips begin. It is helpful to know the area well. Even if you do not, your public library can provide everything you need for trip planning. Choose a couple of destinations and talk with your group members to see if they have connections to some of your proposed destinations. A drive through an old neighborhood, past a school or place of work can be a tremendous lift for nursing home residents, a reminder that they, too, are part of the real world.

Create a mini-assessment with these questions:

- Where did you live and what do you remember about where you lived?

- What is your favorite landmark in this city?

- Your favorite public park?

- Where is your favorite place to go and why?

- Where did you shop?

- What school did you attend? Your children?

- Did you participate in any sports? If so, where?

- Did you go downtown? Where?

- Favorite corner store?

- Favorite hangout?

Chapter Five

Memory Lane is exclusively for the high-cognitive resident. However, any bus trip can be beneficial for both the low-cognitive resident and the Alzheimer's resident. Normalization, simply stated, means providing situations for the people inside the facility similar to those they would experience living on the outside. Participating in an outing to a restaurant allows the residents to experience something they have been familiar with in their past lives. Going to pubs, corner bars, and evening outings also allow for remembering good times.

> *Steve was a wheelchair-bound, 80-year-old retired factory worker. He had ten children but rarely any visitors. He would often reminisce about his 40 years at the same job, working his way from assembly line to head foreman. This was a triumph for Steve and he was proud of it. Needless to say, our trip to the 'factory' and our introduction of Steve to the current employees taking a 'smoke break' was a moment he'll never forget.*

Today's News

Today's News is for the very cognitive and involved resident. This is a challenging and thought-provoking group. The key to this group's success is to have a facilitator that is knowledgeable about current events and public speaking. The group meets weekly and reviews the local newspaper or a magazine chosen by the group. The highlights of the week are discussed. Opinions are shared. Moderating the discussion requires a diplomatic facilitator, someone who is comfortable with handling differences, and tolerant of everyone's beliefs. Understanding the political climate is very important for the facilitator. All it takes is a little preparation or research done on the Internet or at your local library.

Goal: To provide an opportunity for the residents to be aware and informed about current events and affairs of the country, state and city.

Objectives:

- Keep residents up-to-date on current and national affairs;

- Stimulate residents to discussion and well-mannered controversy; and

- Help residents be open and challenging about others' opinions and thoughts.

Group Content and Setup

This group can take many turns. The group will lead you to where it wants to be. Field trips are a great adjunct to the discussions. It has been interesting to visit places that have been discussed as a group, and to see changes in the city's landscape that have been reported in the newspaper. Your group may decide to study an issue in-depth, and become involved by writing to government representatives. Let the group choose its own direction, being very careful no hostility comes from an honest difference of opinion.

> *When I moderated a Today's News group in Arizona, the group developed a keen interest in the stock market. We began by choosing ten stocks to follow, each resident choosing a stock for his or her own reason. Betty's son owned a camera shop, so she chose to watch Polaroid. Others picked stocks from the companies they had*

worked for or makers of their favorite products. The group learned the stock market together. No one became an expert, but we all learned and shared our knowledge. After following the ten stocks for a few months, the group took their interest to the next level, and invested money as a group. With this shift in interest and purpose, I had to start a brand new Today's News group.

The group agenda might go as follows:

- Read the front page of the paper (10 minutes);

- Read one article that a member chooses from a current political magazine (10 minutes);

- Discuss either the headlines or the article (15 minutes); and

- Choose Letters to the Editor to read and discuss (15 minutes).

Once a month, one of my groups invited a speaker from the community to enlighten and challenge the group. We had professors of political science. We had stockbrokers and financial analysts. We invited the CEO of a local power company. The owner of a restaurant chain visited and talked about expansion plans. With all the visitors we received, our Today's News drew some attention. Several of our meetings were highlighted in the local newspaper and covered on local television. "We not only talk about the news," one of my residents said to me, "we *make* the news."

Faith, Hope and Charity

For any resident, being aware of where one is and knowing why one is in a facility can be a very difficult realization. The activity services staff is responsible for providing a stimulating environment. Residents who have some kind of satisfaction in their lives find that their days don't "drag on." Residents who are self-directed and have established leisure activities tend to deal with the nursing home placement more effectively than those with nothing to do or those without personal projects or hobbies.

Faith, Hope and Charity is ideal for the resident without a hobby, but with some religious affiliations and an enjoyment of Bible reading. This group of oriented residents meets weekly to help organize volunteer pastors and religious groups to visit the nursing home. The primary focus is to ensure that residents with religious interests have their spiritual needs met on a regular basis. This group's major intent is to attend to the religious needs of all the residents.

> *Andrew had been an elder in his church for over 40 years. He knew and loved the Bible. He could sit for hours discussing parables and stories from the Bible. He showed immediate interest in Faith, Hope and Charity and helped me organize the group. After months of building a cohesive and productive group, Andy asked if he could lead and facilitate the group on his own. Andy blossomed in his new role. He was so engrossed in his responsibility, he took religious courses at the local community college. After four years of dedication to Faith, Hope and Charity, Andy went to his Lord. In memory, the group changed its name to include his.*

Goal: To meet the spiritual needs of group members.

Objectives:

- Provide empowerment to group members by offering tasks which help them adjust to living a normal life in the facility;

- Provide a deep spiritual opportunity;

- Provide the opportunity to discuss spiritual matters with community leaders; and

- Create a positive church-related program for other residents.

Chapter Five

Group Content and Setup

Faith, Hope and Charity allows the oriented resident to help those who are less capable by working with peers he or she is comfortable with. The group members are able to take on some duties for the activity services staff, who must assess all the residents' spiritual needs. If the facility is blessed with a chaplain, this would be a very appropriate time for the chaplain to be involved. The spiritual assessment can be the link—it is an easy tool for the residents in the group to use for an introductory meeting with nonmember residents. The assessment should be brief and simple, something your group members can complete with training.

Are you a spiritual person?	Yes No
If yes, what religion do you practice?	_____
Do you find strength in the Bible?	Yes No
If yes, how often do you read it?	Daily/weekly/monthly/ I would like to be read to.

Once spiritual assessments have been conducted, the facilitator is ready to begin setting specific goals for this therapeutic group. Allow the group members to take part in creating an assessment that works for your facility. The more suggestions you act upon, the more they will feel empowered and in control of their group.

Supplies needed:

- Weekly meeting schedule;

- Telephone and telephone book, or a list of churches, synagogues and temples in the area;

- List of all religious affiliations of all the residents; and

- List of all the ongoing religious programs offered at the facility.

It is effective to have a small group, but the therapeutic value of this group is extensive. The group is success oriented. The residents become integrated with the community by meeting with the clergy of the area. They can establish a volunteer group that visits the facility, and may go as far as to visit the various churches in the area.

This group can arrange visits from the surrounding churches for residents who are lonely or isolated. The oriented residents can visit new residents, to determine if they would like to participate in a religious program or have a visitor from the church come and see them. Some group members will not be interested in doing this. Those that are interested can also be involved with the One-On-One room visit program described earlier in this chapter. For those who are not interested in visiting, doing the research allows them to feel important, needed and worthwhile while staying in their own comfort zone.

If a facility is fortunate enough to have a chaplain on its staff, then the chaplain should lead this group. If not, the hospices involved with the facility will have chaplains who might be interested in Bible study groups or working with groups such as Faith, Hope and Charity. The agenda for the group meetings should be very clear and should follow the same structure every week.

This group's agenda might go as follows:

1. Opening prayer;

2. Review of religious groups participating in facility. This should be listed on a poster board that can be brought weekly to the meeting. Any changes or relocation of programs can be announced at this time (5 minutes);

3. Review of new residents who have shown an interest in participating in a religious group (2–10 minutes);

4. Report by group members who have visited new residents (5–10 minutes);

5. Need for new spiritually oriented groups and inviting new residents to established groups (2 minutes);

6. Telephone calls or research time for new volunteers. Confirming volunteers who are presently involved in facility (5–10 minutes);

7. Bible study time, if the group would like to do personal growth (5–10 minutes); and

8. Wrap up and scheduling for the next meeting, as well as work to do throughout the week (3–10 minutes).

Chapter Five

Activities during the week might include:

- Sitting in on Bible studies that are going on;

- Checking to make sure residents are receiving promised visits; and

- Welcoming ministers and volunteers to facility and giving tours.

Two types of weekly sessions can be offered. The shorter version is a half-hour session, used to review spiritual activities in the facility briefly, and to do light Bible study. The longer one-hour version allows the group to take ownership of all religious activities in the facility. This is recommended and might be the final outcome of the shorter group once it is established.

If there is a chaplain or spiritual leader who would take on this group, their participation will be very valuable. The Bible study time could be a half-hour and the planning and facilitating could be a half-hour. Therapeutic groups that provide ownership and require empowerment cannot be rushed. Allow time for the group to bond and form a cohesive unit. The discussion on group therapy (see chapter eight) will help you understand the dynamics of this and other more profound groups. Since your members will, in most cases, have had a lifelong interest in spiritual matters, they are not likely to lose interest in this group. Time is on your side.

Pen Pals

Written communication is fast becoming a lost art. Residents get great satisfaction from receiving a letter in the mail. "But you can't get one if you don't write one," was always my response to the resident who complained of letter isolation. Pen Pals works directly to solve this problem. You will find that if your residents write, they will receive letters. Communication by the written word becomes a revitalized form of communication.

Goal: To create a positive atmosphere based on the group's correspondence.

Objectives:

- Provide an opportunity to communicate to other people in the United States, Canada and possibly even around the world;

- Provide the enjoyment of writing and communicating with others; and

- Establish connections to others via letters and postcards.

Group Content and Setup

This therapeutic group has been very successful in many facilities. There is but one goal at the beginning of this group. The goal of Pen Pals therapeutic group is to have correspondence with all 50 states and the ten provinces in Canada. (It is not as easy as it sounds.) This involves sending a postcard or letter to at least one nursing facility in each state or province, and receiving a reply. It is very easy to establish your criteria for the group. Members must be alert, oriented, and able to hear. It is not mandatory for the resident to write; often one member will do all the writing for a meeting. Members must have an interest in writing or enjoy receiving letters. This is established at the time of the initial assessment.

It is crucial to establish a routine in the writing of the letters. The weekly meeting

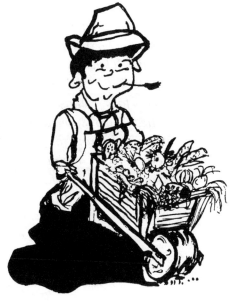

time and day, as in all therapeutic groups, must be adhered to and established at the beginning of the group. The structure of the half-hour meeting is also very important. It is easy to obtain a list of facilities interested in exchanging letters. Refer to trade journals and newsletters. Get a large map of the United States or North America, depending on your group's personal goals, and mount it on a corkboard. The facilitator should have two or three names of facilities prior to beginning each meeting. Every time you send out a letter, place a flag pin where the letter is headed. Every time the group receives a letter, put a check mark on the flag. It is important to stay organized with the group as to the whereabouts of the letters. It has also been a favorite pastime for some Pen Pals groups to decorate letters and envelopes and sell them to make money for postage and paper. The group then becomes self-sufficient.

The routine is weekly and lasts no longer than 30 minutes. The letters are sent out and answered as they arrive. One member of the group should read them and another can pen a reply. At the beginning of the group it is recommended to write the letter as a group. This one letter can be used and recopied as you see fit. A good introductory letter can be used as the first letter you send out to all fifty states. Once the letters start coming in, it might be just as rewarding to give the letters to group members to respond on their own. The members tend to identify strongly with their group as they constantly receive letters and mark states on their map. Once you have achieved some results, display the map in a public area between meetings.

Mamie, a 90-year-old retired schoolteacher, loved the idea of writing letters. She insisted on being the secretary of our Pen Pal group in Florida. The Pen Pal group consisted of seven residents: two schoolteachers, a librarian, a store owner, a musician and a couple who owned their own business making and selling business cards. It was a wonderful group and they found the task of writing to 50 states and ten provinces exhilarating. Mamie immediately found four friends in four states and asked for nursing homes in their cities. The response was immediate. Mamie received letters within two weeks from all four states. She was thrilled. She brought the letters to the resident council meeting and was congratulated in front of the entire facility. Mamie never forgot that overwhelming response both from the distant facilities and from her fellow residents. She took the role of secretary seriously, and kept it through her final days with us.

Hospitality Club

Margaret was always very active in her church. She did not have many physical limitations, but since her husband was in the facility she felt she had to stay to be near him. He was in the second or third stage of Alzheimer's disease and had little recollection of his wife. Margaret had two beautiful daughters who were also very involved in the facility. Her daughters carried on their mother's interest in the community and often volunteered at the facility. Margaret just didn't get too involved in anything and began to get more and more depressed. One day I went to Margaret and asked her to help me welcome visitors into our fine facility. She said, "What on earth for?" I just said I needed help for the afternoon, and she was the one that I wanted to help me. With a little hesitation she agreed.

She was exceptional, telling all the visitors about the facility and showing them exactly where they needed to go. Margaret really was a natural. The next time we asked Margaret to welcome visitors was for our Mother's Day Tea. She was given a corsage and sat at the entrance welcoming everyone and saying, "Welcome to my home." I knew after this experience, she had filled the hole that had been empty for a long time.

Goal: To provide an avenue for residents to play an active role in the spirit of the facility.

Objectives:

- Increase residents' interest in socializing with other residents and visitors;

- Create an environment of friendship and camaraderie;

- Provide opportunities to be leaders in your facility;

- Offer an avenue for residents to play an important and needed role; and

- Provide an opportunity for residents who enjoyed volunteer work in the past.

Chapter Five

Group Content and Setup

The Hospitality Club meets on a weekly or biweekly basis for a half-hour. The residents this group attracts are the most social, outgoing people in the facility. Their role is very front and center. They are your public relations officers.
Residents who seem to benefit with this group are:

- Those active and involved with the day-to-day life of the facility. This could be the only therapeutic group in which they need to be involved.

- Residents who sit in the lobby and are not involved in many other activities.

- Officers of the resident council.

- The self-directed resident who often refuses to attend "nursing home" activities.

- Residents who are involved in their own personal care and take pride in how they look every day.

Channeling the resident who might otherwise complain puts his or her energies into a constructive mode. This must be carefully monitored, since residents can easily broadcast negatives about your facility. A positive resident, involved in training, can redirect their complaints and use their energies in a valuable way.

Duties of the Participants:

Delivering Birthday Cards—Compile, sign, and deliver all the birthday cards in the facility. When the group gets together, the cards are signed by all of the members and then delivered by a group member. Allocating responsibilities in this group is important. Members are interested in being given responsibilities, and in doing things that are important and needed. The facilitator can hand out the cards a month in advance with the name, room number and birthday of the resident on the outside of the card and ask each member of the group to deliver their cards in a timely fashion. It is totally acceptable for the facilitator to accompany the group member delivering the cards.

Sending Get-Well Cards—Sign and send get-well cards for the residents in the hospital. The facilitator may need to help get addresses, but the group should be able to handle everything else.

Visiting the Sick and Sad—The group members can decide on their visiting schedules. Do they visit residents who are more depressed than normal? Do they visit residents who are ill and just returned from the hospital? Do they visit residents who just lost a roommate or a loved one? Your group members will have to decide on their own criteria for visiting. This is also done specifically by the One-On-One group described in this chapter. The major difference is that these visits are short-term and not planned with too many specific goals and objectives. Depression and dealing with personal issues is a sensitive area due to the regulations on confidentiality. You are permitted to say, "Margaret, Angela is sad to-day, would you mind stopping in and saying 'Hello.'" But, to keep con-versations from becoming too intense, you may want to recommend visits last less than five minutes.

Official Public Relations Representative—Many special events are held at your facility. This group will officially greet all the visitors at the door and direct them to the event. Family Night and National Nursing Home Week events have proven to be a very positive experience for the Hospitality Club members.

Official Greeters—Do you put together a schedule for the members to fol-low on welcoming visitors, family and friends into the facility? This again is the facilitator's call. The group I have been involved with de-cided no schedule was necessary. They just wore their nametags when they were out in the hall and entryway.

> *Peter had lived at the facility for over five years and he was a permanent fixture in the lobby. Peter was known by everyone, from families to the Federal Express driver to the food-and-supplies delivery men. He waved and updated the regulars on baseball scores. Everyone smiled and welcomed his kindness and friendli-ness. Peter was asked to join the Hospitality Club. At first, he said he couldn't offer anything to the group. After a few more requests, he attended. Peter became the president of the club and now*

continues his welcoming style, proudly wearing his "Resident Greeter" Hospitality Club nametag. Incidentally, Peter never missed a meeting after he joined.

Outline for Group

As mentioned before, it is wise to stay within a half-hour limit for meetings. It is also advisable to stick to an agenda for each meeting. This does not allow time for inappropriate discussion. A possible agenda would be:

1. Opening: Ask a member of the group to choose a poem and read it to the group;

2. Read the prepared agenda to the group and ask for any additions or corrections;

3. Review past events and ask for discussion;

4. Review past visits and share feelings and thoughts on the visits;

5. Invite a member of the staff to come in to discuss special events where hospitality will be important;

6. Sign cards; and

7. Discuss upcoming events and activities.

A Special Friend—An Intergenerational Connection

This is not a new concept or a new group, but it is too often neglected in a nursing home. This is an easy group to facilitate, but a more complex group to plan and implement.

Goal: To connect with younger people in the community.

Objectives:

- Provide an opportunity to meet and get to know new people in the community;

- Provide an avenue to be with children and youth; and

- Provide grandparents to a grandparent-less child and vice versa.

The first step in planning an intergenerational group in a nursing home is to establish a relationship with neighborhood elementary schools. A letter of introduction to the principal does this. Explain the importance of children and older adults being in each other's lives. Mention the value of children learning about life in a nursing home. Explain that children can get their first experience in community service, and learn about their community through visiting your facility. This letter should ask for a commitment on the part of the school to visiting or being visited every month of the school year. Commitment is crucial for this program to work. Consistency makes it a meaningful part of the residents' lives and the children's lives.

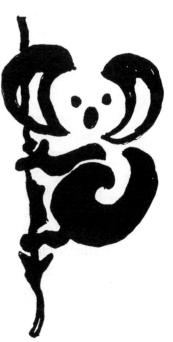

Once a relationship is established with the principal, and a commitment agreed upon for regular visits, the planning of the program needs the involvement of the activity services staff and the teacher who will be bringing the children. Simple ideas work best for this program. Crafts, songs and games are uncomplicated and easy for all ages. On one occasion, we invited a craft teacher who taught stamp art. We used a large roll of newsprint (available from the local newspaper) and the children and residents created a scene on the newsprint of the circus that was in town for the week.

77

It was enormously successful for both age groups. The local supermarket agreed to hang the poster in a prominent spot for the whole community to enjoy. The children, the residents, the community, and especially our public relations director, were all thrilled with this project.

Other ideas that have been successful in intergenerational programming:

- *Simple seasonal crafts:* Table decorations, door decorations, and cards.

- *Singing by either group:* This is very successful when local nursery schools and day-care centers are invited. It is more of a special event than a regular part of the program. The more the children perform in front of the residents, the more comfortable the children will feel with them.

- *Seasonal or holiday baking.*

- *Life Stories:* This program was initiated with the local high school. A high-school English class was in search of a project. Life Stories were suggested to their teacher. A group of students interviewed a variety of residents who wanted to participate and discuss their lives and their interests. The students designed a group of questions with help from the activity services director. The students asked the same questions of twenty residents, then made a life story of their answers. The stories were then collated and placed into a book. The book was given to all the residents involved and sold at the high school craft fair.

- *Wheelchair Wash-a-thon:* This was initiated by the activity services director due to the lack of evening employees available to clean wheelchairs. A junior high-school home economics class was looking for a community service project, and agreed to participate. The Wash-a-thon was held indoors (due to cold weather) in the various shower and bathing rooms. All the supplies were available from the housekeeping department. The students, mostly boys, were enthusiastic and involved. They had personal contact with residents as they went to get the wheelchairs and return them to their owners. This was a successful biannual program.

- *Costume making:* This works well during festive times of year such as for Halloween and for theme days. The group gets together to try on hats and decorate them together. The laughter and fun can be heard throughout the halls.

- *Outings to schools:* We have had very successful outings to plays and choir performances. But our most popular event is when the residents visit the school during lunch and share lunch with the students in the cafeteria. This is not recommended for the Alzheimer's resident, but is very positive for the more oriented resident.

- *Church groups:* Many local churches have youth groups that enjoy community service. There is not one activity services director reading this that has not received a phone call around the Christmas holiday season with an offer of carolers coming to sing. The policy that I have established wherever I work is as follows: "We appreciate the fact that you would like to sing to our residents during this festive time of year. We have a number of carolers during this time and if your group will commit to three other times during the year, you are welcome to come in December." The response from the church groups has always been overwhelming. During one call, the activity services staff booked a group for four times during the year. The groups react with enthusiasm and astonishment. They appreciate the residents' need for visitors, but usually have never realized that the need is so great. We are teaching the children that although Christmas is important, February and September can also be lonely months.

- *Extracurricular high-school groups:* If you need a group of young people for a specific purpose, go to the coach of the basketball team or debating team and suggest a single project, something brief, yet vital to your programming. This is often very effective. As you can see, necessity will often provide an opportunity for intergenerational experiences. Once your initial contacts are made, teachers and school administrators do much of the planning and organizing. This is an area of activity that can be started up easily, and tends to keep going on its own momentum.

Chapter Five

The call came as a bit of a surprise. Like many others, our facility is a polling place. The local sponsors of Kids Vote wanted to put their program in place at the facility, so children could vote when they came to the polls with their parents. Of course, it would take some work. Kids Vote wanted staff members to help the kids as they came in to vote. "Well," I asked, "How about some of our residents doing that?" The Kids Vote representative never had anyone suggest this, and seemed somewhat skeptical. "Come to a meeting of the Hospitality Club, and decide for yourself," I offered. After that, it was a done deal. One of our club members had been a kindergarten teacher for almost 50 years. Others members had taught, volunteered, or worked with children. All had children and grandchildren of their own. The sponsors fell in love with our residents, and the program was fabulous for everyone involved. It was also an opportunity for activity services to be the public relations arm of our facility, and our residents were delighted with the newspaper and television coverage they got. So was our administrator.

Spelling Bee

This therapeutic group is designed for a very specific group of residents. When I started in my most recent directorship, I found that our residents had been enjoying spelling on a weekly basis for many years. The structure of the group, however, was loosely defined. The nurse's aides would bring any resident into the group as part of the morning program routine. The residents who could not spell simple words or could not understand the rules of the spelling bee irritated the advanced spellers. This forced the activity services staff to question the goals and purpose of the group. It was an interesting exercise in designing a therapeutic group.

Goals: To provide a stimulating environment for residents to maintain or develop mental abilities.

Objectives:

- Offer a feeling of success in a group environment;

- Improve spelling skills;

- Learn new words;

- Use words in a sentence;

- Learn the official rules and regulations of a spelling bee; and

- Provide an opportunity for competition on a friendly and cooperative basis.

In examining these objectives, I concluded that we had a therapeutic group that worked for high-functioning residents only. Once your activity service staff understands what they are trying to achieve, they are more likely to succeed.

When you know how specific your group needs to be, you are able to select programs appropriate to the needs of the remaining residents. Once we discovered that the spelling bee was specifically for the high-functioning resident, we were able to identify others who enjoyed morning programs, and create programming for the group that had not been participating.

You might want to offer several levels of spelling bee. The words and rules can be made simpler for a lower functioning group. But far more likely, another therapeutic group would work for the residents who are not able to participate. Spell and Tell, as described in chapter four, is a group for low-cognitive residents that offers a variation on Spelling Bee. This could be an appropriate choice for another group during that same time period.

The spelling bee group blossomed. The activity services staff was very detailed in the rules and regulations for the group. The group responded in kind, demanding we use "official" spelling bee rules, which were researched and put in place.

Spelling Bee Rules (nursing home version additions):

- All participants must pronounce, spell, and pronounce again each word they are given;

- A proper noun may be given and the speller will have to start the spelling of the word with "capital;" and

- Spellers will be given one extra chance to spell a word correctly.

It is good to post these rules and review them. It helps to make a sign on poster board to be placed as a reminder to contestants: "Pronounce, Spell, Pronounce" and a piece of paper in front of each of the spellers with this same reminder.

"Pronounce, Spell, Pronounce" was the mantra I kept hearing in the hall-ways. The residents involved practiced instinctively as they went to dinner. This got me thinking. These residents are dedicated, and need to show the world their knowledge and commitment to this group and to their craft. If this is true in my facility, then other facilities must have residents equally interested in words and competition. I sent out a letter (see sample on page 83) and invited neighboring facilities to join us for competitions.

The response was overwhelming. Immediately, the calls came in and we decided to invite two facilities every Thursday. It was extremely successful. The most positive part of the events was the involvement of the residents at our facility. They took on their roles as host and hostess with dignity. They welcomed the visiting facilities and served them hospitably. Without a doubt, they were welcoming their new friends into their home. The group continues today and our team still discusses the wonderful visitors they had from and around the Cincinnati area.

Date

Dear Activity Director,

We, at the <u>Facility Name</u>, would like to invite your residents to one of our spelling bee competitions. We are having a spelling bee competition the third Thursday of every month, beginning in September. We are looking for the ten best spellers from your facility. By April, we will have the top spellers organized and ready for the Championship Game to be held during National Nursing Home Week.

We are really excited about extending this invitation to you. Just call us and choose the month that would work best for you. The monthly competitions will be held in the atrium at <u>time or day</u>. We will provide lemonade, cookies, and time to socialize and meet new friends.

We hope this idea works for you—please do not hesitate to call and book your spelling bee competition date.

Looking forward to hearing from you.

Sincerely,

<u>Signature</u>

Ruth was a brand-new resident. She asked about the upcoming spelling bee competition. "I love to spell," she exclaimed. "I won my grade three spelling bee some 60 years ago." She continued, "The winners of the spelling bee were invited to hear a guest speaker at the university several hours distant." Her parents were hesitant to allow her to go on the trip, but finally agreed. Ruth will never forget her trip to hear Helen Keller's speech. Ruth ended up winning the second spelling bee of her lifetime.

Interest-Based Groups

Lucille was a woman who never married. She worked in the post office before retirement, and she always had animals in her life. She enjoyed dogs mostly. She came to the facility in the later stages of Alzheimer's, still able to walk but not able to speak coherently. Her assessment was completed appropriately and accurately. Her family was involved with her assessment and told activity services staff of her love for animals.

Ethel had been married. She never had children, but always had two or more dogs in her home. These two ladies met during Puppy Pals. The group met to discuss and be with animals and share their love of animals. Ethel was always talkative, and always sat beside Lucille during the group. One day Ethel was holding Hershey, a miniature dachshund, and passed her to Lucille. Ethel said how cute the dog was and asked Lucille if she ever had a dog like this. Lucille looked up and straight at Ethel and said, "Yes, her name was Frieda." This breakthrough brought Ethel and Lucille even closer. Ethel ended up visiting Lucille (within the One-On-One therapeutic group) and they became good friends. And yes, Lucille really did have a Frieda in her life.

Chapter Six

Groups discussed in this chapter—

- Welcome Club

- Let's Talk Dirt

- A Show of Hands

- Puppy Pals

- Music in Motion

- Beauty Spot

- Sports Stuff

- Sit and Be Fit

- Family Tea Hour

- Facility Chorus

We have talked about groups for residents with high and low cognitive levels. There are many groups that have no prerequisite of cognitive level. These groups are called interest-based groups. Although they have therapeutic value, these groups are aimed strictly at the interests of the resident. The groups must be run with flexibility in their planning and implementation to allow any and all interested residents the opportunity to participate. Placement in these groups is based on the assessment of the resident, not their cognitive level as in other groups we have discussed. When a resident is not able to verbalize his past interests, an assessment from a family member will be enough to allow proper placement in these groups.

The key to successful placement in these groups is the participants' interest level, not the level of ability or skills. Residents participate in interest-based groups for a definite purpose. Interest-based groups center on what participants have done all their life, what is needed to make them feel at home, and what provides them with comfortable surroundings. The goals can be simple and the objectives brief.

As they participate, look for definite results. The goals we are trying to attain for each resident are different. Results can vary according to each individual's abilities. The low cognitive residents' goals would focus on hand-eye coordination and length of stay in the group. As for the higher cognitive resident, the goal would be leadership, socialization, and improving his or her skills. The groups are designed to create a comfort level. That comfort level should be noted and documented as results are seen.

These groups have been used before, but need to have systems established for facilitation and presentation. Most interest-based groups last between 30 and 60 minutes due to lengthy setup and preparation. Groups should have six to eight members unless otherwise stated. Interest-based groups should be run weekly, just like the groups described in other sections of this book.

The basis and goals of the groups are preestablished, but flexibility and adaptability are vital to make these groups work. The criteria for admission to the group is simply the interest and past lifestyle choices of the resident. The groups tend to lend themselves to the participants. Often the group's content will change as membership changes. It is helpful to follow the guidelines in this chapter with participants' abilities in mind at all times.

Remember, these interest-based groups have no prerequisite of cognitive level. Both high-functioning and low-functioning residents can participate as long as they feel comfortable together.

Chapter Six

Welcome Club

No matter what a person's age is, change is unsettling and moving is scary. Welcome Club was established to ease fears during the adjustment period for a new resident. The move to the nursing home could be the most traumatic event in the life of an individual. Not only moving itself, but also losing possessions and independence need to be faced squarely. So many times a new resident has no one to talk to about these drastic changes. Welcome Club offers an outstretched hand and provides comfort to the incoming resident.

Goal: To provide appropriate information for the new resident.

Objectives:

- Get to know the facility as a whole and understand available staff and services;

- Socialize with other new residents;

- Learn the routine of the facility;

- Learn names of some of the key people involved in the daily care of the resident; and

- Provide an avenue to meet people who share the fears and questions one has when admitted to a nursing home.

As the name implies, the Welcome Club provides an opportunity for the new resident to learn about the facility. This group meeting gives staff a regular time slot to offer the information new residents need and to introduce them to the workings of the facility. This group consists of five standard sessions. A new resident joins in the group after a week's stay in the facility, and attends for five weeks. The sequence of sessions will vary for participants as residents arrive at different times in the cycle. At the end of five weeks, they will have been through all five programs, and will be ready to integrate into other groups. Sessions are limited to a half-hour each, so participating staff can budget their time. Sessions are held on the same day each week.

Since residents can enter the group at any time, there is no "final meeting" in this group. Sometimes residents have difficulty leaving, because this is their first social contact group and they have a deep connection to it. When the last meeting occurs for a resident, individually review all the opportunities available to him or her in the form of activities and social contacts. If the resident is not ready to move on, invite him or her back for another week. It does not matter if the resident repeats a few weeks until he or she is ready to move on.

Group Content and Setup

The setup of this group must be the same every week, although the location may vary. I recommend having the group meet in a resident's room. This allows the resident to feel like he or she is "entertaining" and receiving people in his or her "home." It provides an ownership that is truly important. Make sure the facilitator asks permission well in advance for the use of a resident's room each week. If that is not possible, a small lounge would be appropriate.

I also recommend that the host or hostess of the group be involved in choosing what food and beverage is to be served. Supply the host with an appropriate menu with a small selection of a variety of foods that are easily prepared by the dietary staff. Our menu includes cookies, fruit, small cakes, pretzels, chips, and beverage choices such as coffee, tea, lemonade and fruit punch. This gives the host responsibility and involvement in the group.

Facilitator's Guidelines

1. **Create an Invitation** to send out to new members or as a reminder for current members. This can be included in the admission package or handed out by activity services.

Welcome to <u>Facility Name</u>

Join the Welcome Club and learn more about <u>Facility Name</u>.

We meet <u>Day of the Week</u> at <u>time</u>
in the <u>location</u>.

For more information contact the
Activity Services Department.

---

2. **Conducting the Group**

a. **Welcome to Group (2 minutes).** Set a climate of acceptance. Mention the name of the facility and your name and position. Tell the new residents that the group lasts for five weeks and will answer their questions about the facility. Personally welcome any new members starting this week. Explain that residents can begin at any time during the five weeks, and they are always welcome in the Welcome Club.

b. **Introductions and Nametags (5 minutes).** Assign a resident to write and hand out nametags. At this time allow each resident to introduce himself or herself, or help introduce the resident who is unable to introduce himself or herself. Allow time for the resident to speak about themselves at this time.

c. **Refreshments (3 minutes).** The host or hostess is usually the person who serves the snack. It is a nice touch to use regular glasses and plates.

d. **Poem (1 minute).** The facilitator can choose a poem. Usually the facilitator asks a resident to read the poem. This poem can be repeated from one week to the next, or can even be a standard that is always used. Select a short, simple, "feel good" poem, and reproduce it in large type for easy reading. Ask participants to recommend poetry to be read at the next meeting of the group.

e. **Discussion of Poems (2 minutes).** Often the poem provides an avenue for discussion. Many people enjoy listening to poems. If it is seasonal or personal, allow time for members to say a few words.

f. **Discussion of Session Topics (15 minutes).** Topics vary from session to session. Detailed topic notes follow.

g. **Closure and Thanks (2 minutes).** Announce when the next meeting will be. Ask for a volunteer host or hostess for the next meeting, perhaps saying, "It was so wonderful meeting in Joanne's room; would you like us to come back, or would you rather someone else host our next meeting?" Often the residents do not remember scheduled meetings, so a small invitation to remind them the day before is often helpful.

Session Topics

Session #1—Welcome to the Facility

The brand-new resident is going to have many questions about his or her new environment. He or she will be uncertain about the many adjustments he or she will have to make. This welcome session provides answers to questions like this:

- Where do I voice complaints? (Make it clear that *all* of your staff are willing to help them solve problems. Make that a policy, not just a slogan.)

- What does the call light mean? How and why would I use the call light?

- What is a nurse's aide, and what does he or she do?

- What about meals? Visiting hours? Activities?

Introduce one or two nurse's aides, and ask them to tell a little about themselves. Give the incoming resident the view that the nurse's aides are real people, as well as employees of the facility. If the resident is not verbal, see if a family member can sit in on this session, and help with communication.

The nurse's aide is an integral part of the workings of the facility. He or she is the front-line staff. No one is as close to the resident as a the nurse's aide. Allow him or her to become personal to the resident. Help him or her establish a relationship that is positive and open with the resident.

This is also an appropriate time to discuss the other departments that the resident might encounter. Discuss the possibility of having a light bulb burn out and requiring the help of the maintenance department. Inform the resident of the name of the director of maintenance and his or her staff and the hours they are usually in the building. Inform the resident that anyone in the department could come to his or her room and fix the light bulb.

The relationship of the resident and the housekeeping department is also crucial. Often the housekeepers know more personal information about the resident than anyone else in the facility does. They are often the residents' choice in whom to confide. Discuss their role and their importance to the resident, and any other pertinent staff that you feel could be of value to the resident. All facilities are slightly different in the roles of the departments. Make sure the roles are spelled out and everyone understands.

Session #2

Now we start dealing with resident's personal issues, particularly their reaction to nursing home placement. For this session, you should invite the social services staff to join you. The facilitator is not to answer the profound questions. His or her job is to channel the questions to the correct person.

The facilitator might begin the discussion period with questions such as:

- How do you feel about being here?

- How are things different for you?

- Are you comfortable here?

- Would you like to meet more people?

- Who have you met?

- Who do you remember by name?

- What does that person do?

It is a good idea to start a homework-type game, asking each resident to remember one name of another resident or staff member, and bring it back to the following meetings. This is a good memory game and a way to get conversation started for the new resident.

Session #3

Talk in more depth about the adjustments the residents will need to make, and adjustments the facility can make for their benefit in this session. This session should also include introductions of the director of nursing and the nursing staff involved in direct care of the residents.

Topics might include:

- What the residents left behind.

- What they miss about their former surroundings.

- What does it mean to the residents to be in a nursing home?

- How can the staff make the transition smoother?

- What would make the new resident's stay more comfortable?

- If the residents could change three things in this nursing home, what would they be?

- How would you change them?

Do not let the residents use this group as a complaint forum. Allow them the opportunity to solve problems for themselves. If a resident has a complaint, use it as a catalyst for finding a solution when necessary.

You should also discuss the duties of the nurses and their medication regime, such as the routine for medication carts and the duties involved in passing medications.

Session #4

This session is a listening session more than a teaching session. We discuss the new resident's former lifestyle. This is a great opportunity for the facilitator to really find out about the resident. The facilitator can make it a discussion of things they remember. This is often a productive meeting for activity services staff, as they can form an assessment and decide which therapeutic groups the resident will be involved in after they finish with Welcome Club.

Topics can include:

• What did your job mean to you?

• What was your home like?

• What did you do before you retired? When and how did you retire?

• How involved were you in the church and community?

• What were your favorite hobbies and activities?

• Tell the group about your family.

Session #5

This becomes the "commercial" for the activity department. During this meeting the group examines the activity calendar. It is great fun to review all the activities available for the residents.

The facilitator will go through the calendar of events, day-by-day for a week, review the therapeutic groups and the diversionary activities, and then highlight the special events for the month. Have residents who have started getting involved in groups and activities share their experiences. Make sure the facilitator is familiar with all the available groups, and can guide residents toward appropriate groups to meet their needs. Remember, this is not always the last session for a given resident, but it is always an important one for activity services.

Chapter Six

Summary

This group meets for five weeks to provide an overview of the facility and everything it has to offer the resident. The criteria for involvement is simple. All residents who have been in the facility for one week should be invited to attend the next scheduled meeting. It is wise to allow the residents time to get adjusted to their new routine and schedule, since this is a small group setting which could make them feel uncomfortable. They should, of course, be invited to diversionary activities from their first day in the facility. Welcome Club can be the first connection a resident needs to feel like he or she belongs to a facility.

> Jeane was a "wanderer." She walked day and night, and responded to pleasantries in a rather offhanded way. Jeane did not get involved in any diversionary activities because her attention span would not permit it. She might stay for musical entertainment, but it was rare. Jeane was asked if she would like to be the hostess for the Welcome Club. She said she was very busy, but she would try. That afternoon, Kim brought the snacks she had chosen and helped her set up. Jeane was apprehensive but stayed with Kim as she arranged the chairs and the space to fit the members in Jeane's room.
>
> During the meeting Kim asked Jeane to write the nametags and, as it turned out, Jeane had beautiful penmanship. She wrote the nametags beautifully. Jeane continued to write and she asked if she could take the minutes to the meeting and wrote everything the facilitator asked her to write. We had found a niche for Jeane. Kim ended the meeting and told several people of Jeane's newfound skill. Jeane now writes the minutes to nurses' meetings, social service meetings, dietary meetings, and housekeeping meetings. She is kept busy much of the day. She found a place to be useful through the Welcome Club.

Let's Talk Dirt

Gardening groups are widespread in nursing homes. Horticulture therapy is popular among those who work with the aged. There is so much that can be done with earth and imagination. This group will care for plants on an ongoing basis. It is recommended that they have good use of their hands and good hand-eye coordination to plant by themselves. It helps to be able to discuss different topics, especially past gardening experience. Group members need a love of gardening.

Goal: To provide residents with hands-on experience with dirt and gardening.

Objectives:

- Provide an opportunity to use a variety of gardening hand tools;

- Provide an opportunity to share the experience of gardening; and

- To verbalize past interest and love for gardening.

Group Content and Setup

Like many interest-based therapeutic groups, the group leader must understand his or her members and appreciate their varying levels of cognitive ability. This simply means that a gardening program must have tasks available at a variety of skill levels. The program must meet the need for challenge and stimulation of both the oriented gardener and the Alzheimer's resident who has had plants all of his or her life. How do you develop a program that suits the needs of all the different members of the group? The answer to this question will change as group membership changes. Understanding your membership is not difficult. Basically, everyone wants to be with other people that appreciate him or her. This program, as all other interest-based groups, allows the resident one simple comfort: Everyone there enjoys the experience they are sharing.

> *Angela was a very physically active resident, able to walk around the facility. Angela had serious memory problems, and was unable to continue living at home. One of her true joys was raking and taking care of her garden. We learned this during our talks with her in Welcome Club. She was permanently placed in a room with a*

view of the courtyard. She loved to watch the birds, to walk around the courtyard and examine her work. Angela would water her entire garden every day with a watering can. We had a dry, hot summer and she was happy as she could be watering her beans, tomatoes and flowers. Angela often became agitated with her roommate and with her surroundings, but all we had to do to calm her was redirect her into her garden. It was her sanctuary. Her love and devotion to this courtyard garden led to an extensive garden project involving Angela, activity services staff, numerous volunteers, and other residents.

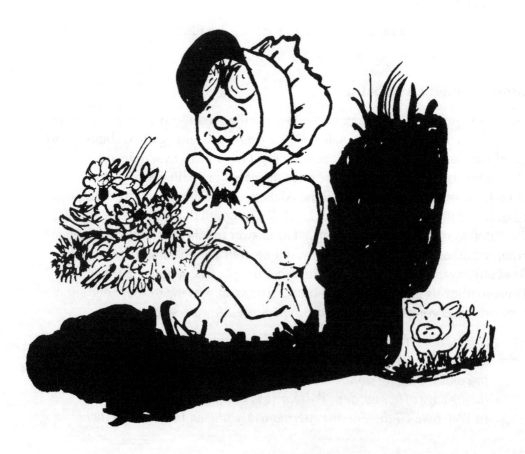

A Show of Hands

Arts and crafts are widely used in nursing facilities. Using the abilities of each interested resident makes this common activity part of the "therapeutic group" theme of this book. Participants should have reasonably good eyesight and dexterity, and past interests in art, graphics, crafts or hobbies. It helps if the group leader has some experience and interest in art. Through research, a fresh flow of ideas and inexpensive materials can be generated. Materials and supplies might include knitting needles, crochet, cross-stitch, crayons, markers, chalk, pencils, charcoal, brushes, paints of various types, paper and canvas, stained glass, glue, scissors, flower arranging, ceramics and pottery.

Goal: To provide residents with hands-on experience with arts and crafts.

Objectives:

- Provide an opportunity for residents to communicate through the medium of art;

- Allow residents to try different techniques to get closer to their feelings; and

- Remind participants of past artistic experiences.

Group Content and Setup

There are so many talented people in this world. You have a number of them right in the palm of your hand. To really use the abilities of your residents is a gift in itself. Using one's own artistic talent can be a wonderful experience.

When you involve the community, particularly young people, you can really make a difference for all involved by helping residents feel closer to the community beyond the nursing home. Begin by inviting neighboring schools to take part in an art show sponsored by your facility. Show of Hands members can share responsibility for the art show. There are many jobs available. The responsibilities can be adjusted to meet the abilities of your membership.

Chapter Six

How to Set Up an Art Contest and Exhibit for Your Facility

Preparations:

1. Prepare a letter to be sent to art teachers at your local elementary and high schools. Send letters at the beginning of the school year to allow teachers to prepare for the theme, and put the dates on the schedule. Letters can be written, stamped and sent by members of the group. One group chose National Nursing Home Week for the show, and used its theme for that year's art competition.

2. Follow up by phone within a week or so to confirm involvement in the show. A member of one Show of Hands group had a phone in her room and called all the schools to determine their interest level.

3. Distribute entry forms with rules and regulations to the participating schools two months before National Nursing Home Week. (See Appendix B for a sample entry form.) Collect artwork during the week prior to the show. Typically, the group I work with will receive artwork the Friday prior to the week of the show, hang it for judging on Sunday, and have an awards ceremony Tuesday evening.

4. Select judges from the community. The judges meet before the exhibit is open to the public. Winning participants should be told prior to the exhibit. Extend a special individual invitation to artist and family of winning entries. The artwork should be judged in categories and by age group.

5. Label all artwork with a colored sticker representing each school. Each piece is then numbered in the appropriate order. For example, if a green sticker designates a given school—and the school sends in 15 pieces—its artwork is numbered Green 1 through Green 15. This color-coding makes it easier to get all the art back to the proper teachers at the end of the show. Make sure all pieces are marked with the artists' age groups (for the judges' sake).

6. Send invitations to all participating schools and the local media. This, like many other events, can create good public relations for your facility.

The Week of the Show

7. Conduct an official art show opening with prizes awarded to the winning art entries that evening. The Show of Hands members can welcome all the participants. The group members that I work with have decided that financial prizes should go to art departments and not individuals. We also give art supplies to each winner. A certificate (see Appendix B) should be awarded to every student involved in the exhibit.

8. Prepare a large check to issue to the art teacher and his or her winning students. Announce all winners and show all winning entries in all categories to participating residents and family members.

9. Leave artwork in place for the duration of National Nursing Home Week. Hang the pieces throughout your facility for all the residents to enjoy.

Puppy Pals

There are facilities that totally support canine visitors, others that are negative about the idea, and still others that are apprehensive and disinterested. This group allows you to share a love of animals within your facility. Facilities have different policies regarding pet visits. Research your facility's policies prior to starting this group. Pet visits increase stimulation through contact with the animals and through interaction among residents. Participants can also share and reminisce once each visit is complete.

Goal: To stimulate interaction between residents using animals as a catalyst.

Objectives:

- Provide residents an opportunity to reminisce about their experiences with animals; and

- Provide the opportunity for residents to see, touch and cuddle a variety of animals.

Group Content and Setup

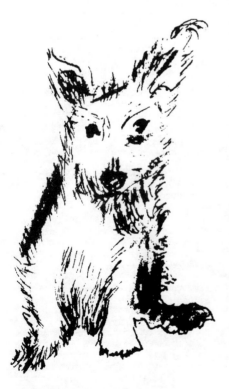

Bring in puppies, kittens, rabbits, reptiles, or anything else that might become available to show to the residents. Have the group sit in a circle and begin with the animal, held by the group leader, in the center. The group leader allows each interested resident to touch or hold the animal, and encourages conversation. Groups with animals produce favorable results because the residents "tune in" to each other and share memories. Many residents like to talk about their former pets. While one resident is speaking, others can enjoy listening, looking at the animals, holding them, or just quietly reminiscing.

Make sure that all participants love animals. Nobody participating should have a fear of animals. It is not the purpose of this group to help residents alleviate their fears in this group setting. When selecting participants, keep in mind that residents who enjoy children will quite often enjoy animals, too. Participants do not need to be verbal, or have perfect vision or hearing.

Keep in mind, while running this widely used activity, that you have goals for the group as a whole and individual goals for participants. The idea is to get residents to talk to each other. The animals are a means to that end.

Many people offer their pets for participation in Puppy Pals. Not all their animals are in fact appropriate for the group. Here's a good method for determining which "volunteers" are appropriate. I have help from two residents who adore animals. The animals (usually dogs) and their owners visit these residents accompanied by an activity services staff member. The residents keep in mind five criteria as they audition the animal:

1. Will the animal act inappropriately if hugged or grabbed by a resident?

2. Does the owner discuss the name and breed of the animal immediately?

3. Does the animal tire easily of being touched and petted?

4. Does the animal shed, salivate, or otherwise appear nervous or scared?

5. Does the owner appear uneasy as the animal is handled?

The criteria are simple and easy for the residents to remember. The resident enjoys the visit tremendously and also revels in the fact that they are "choosing" a pet visitor for the facility. The pet visitor often participates in more than just the half-hour Puppy Pals group. They are given a list of residents who love dogs and are room-bound, or do not participate in groups, and visit their rooms. These visits are recorded in each resident's participation record.

Chapter Six

Music in Motion

Music is the best method of communication with some older adults. I have seen more smiles and laughter surrounding songs and music that any other situation. The residents never complain about your voice or your tone, they just soak it all in. Music is a wonderful catalyst for bringing different residents together. No matter what a resident's cognitive level, often they are able to partake in music programs. Music in Motion can be as challenging as you decide. Invite the residents with a background in music, retired musicians, band leaders, and choir directors. You might be surprised to find out how many of your residents have been involved in music.

You can use such things as:

1. **Resident hand-held instruments:** Provide any instrument from kazoo to cymbals and ask the resident to mimic your movements and create a band.

2. **Band instruments:** Bring in band instruments for the residents to touch and feel. Ask local high-school band members to visit.

3. **Piano:** Challenge the residents to "Name That Tune."

4. **Cassette/CD:** Can the residents identify instruments used in a piece? Similarities between songs (such as themes, words)?

5. **Sing:** Songs from different eras stimulate much discussion and fun.

Goals: To use music as a form of communication and stimulation.

Objectives:

• Increase awareness of the environment through music and musical props;

• Increase residents' range of motion, awareness of space and awareness of their immediate environment;

• Maintain or increase their ability to listen and appreciate music;

• Provide an opportunity to be in a social environment with music;

• Utilize long-term memory to recite songs and tunes; and

• Provide the opportunity to touch and work with a variety of musical instruments.

Group Content and Setup

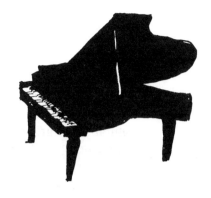

As you have seen the groups mentioned in this chapter are not new to the nursing home industry. There are concepts, though, in each therapeutic group that can help you to *establish a connection* with one or more of your residents.

The use of music is popular in many facilities. The only difference here is this: The activity services staff offers music as a form of therapy rather than straight entertainment. Music is used in a familiar environment to connect with residents in ways they might not normally be reached by staff or other residents. The music is a tool used to unlock memories and stimulate social responses. Feel free to experiment with different kinds of music. Without some variety in

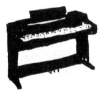

the music you present, residents will tend to fall into a rut, or even fall asleep. The group leader spends the session engaging residents in brief one-on-one conversations centered around the music being presented. Bring in musical instruments for the residents to hold, identify and even play. But remember, the music here is a means to an end, and your goal is to establish connections with and between your residents.

> *Mamie was a frustrated musician. She sang songs from* The Sound of Music *from dawn to dusk. She was very difficult to redirect. She would not sit still for any programs. Judy, our Music in Motion coordinator, decided to put Mamie to the test. She would play a note on the piano and ask if anyone in the room could match it. This seemed like an impossible task. But not for Mamie. She repeated the note in song on the exact pitch. This was indeed a feat. All the facility heard about her ability and she was recognized daily for her accomplishment. She was asked many times to match note for note from a variety of instruments and she could do it every time.*

Chapter Six

Beauty Spot

This type of group activity is conducted in many nursing homes. It is usually called Manicures, and is scheduled every week. The key difference between this therapeutic group and the usual manicures on an activity calendar is the involvement of the resident in the actual programming. It may be helpful to involve an Avon or Mary Kay Cosmetics representative to provide samples and be regular visitors for this group.

Naturally, the group is made up of women. The women in this group have all been very involved in their own personal care issues. There have been residents in this group who have owned beauty parlors, as well as cosmetologists and women who have spent years entertaining and being social. The interest a woman has concerning her skin and her appearance never changes. This is part of a woman's persona. She is either interested in this, or she is not.

Goal: To increase self-confidence and help female residents feel good about themselves.

Objectives:

- Provide a comfortable environment for women to be together;

- Provide an avenue for women to look good and feel great; and

- Provide an environment of relaxation and acceptance of one another.

Group Content and Setup

Assessments will tell you who will be best served by membership in Beauty Spot. Do not allow facilitators to speak amongst themselves. This takes away from the residents' time. It is a poor example for the volunteers, and the residents do not get your undivided attention. This will ostracize the resident immediately. Discuss current events, or items that would be interesting to the residents. The group is much more successful with two or more facilitators. One volunteer or staff member can begin immediately doing manicures as the residents begin to arrive. The music in the background is easy listening music that the residents enjoy and to which they can relate. Small talk and ongoing casual conversation during the session stimulate the group. The facilitators' main goal is to support the formation of friendships between residents as a by-product of their participation. Make sure your facilitator has a topic or two which allows general participation. Repeat statements made by other women for the hard-of-hearing. Do whatever it takes to allow residents to be comfortable with each other.

Beauty Spot can be divided into several subgroups as it unfolds, and it seems to last for hours sometimes. The more volunteers you involve, the more one-on-one interaction can occur. It really makes for a more intimate atmosphere to have a number of small groups of two or three in a larger room. This gives the feeling of a normal beauty parlor atmosphere. The group is structured in such a way that each resident experiences all the subgroups within the larger group.

Group #1—Manicures

This probably occurs in most facilities. It is helpful to have resealable plastic sandwich bags for each resident's personal nail polish. The name of the resident is placed (with marker or nail polish) on the outside of the bag. Keep all of these in a large folder arranged by name. Bowls, towels, moisturizing soap and water are used every week to relax the residents and allow them time to get organized and settled with the entire group.

Group #2—Glamour Gals

Makeup is a large part of Beauty Spot. When two or three women have completed their nail care, the volunteer staff in charge of the makeup gets the group together. It will take about 20 minutes to work with three or four residents. All makeup is already in separate containers. (Try Attends or Wet-Nap boxes.) All residents begin by choosing their own makeup and colors. We have always been able to ask Avon or Mary Kay representatives for extra makeup. We begin by having warm, wet washcloths to wipe the face and the hands. This cleans out the pores and prepares the face for the makeup. The first step would be the moisturizing lotion, followed by the foundation. The group should have a

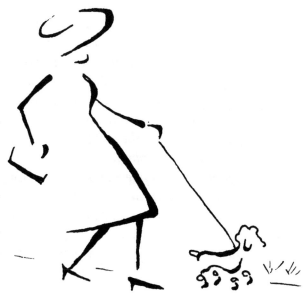

large mirror handy (preferably one that magnifies). Then the eye shadow, eye pencil, lipstick, and blush are all applied. Residents are usually fully aware of their own personal style and routine when it comes to makeup. You might include a brush or comb in each box. Some residents have a real need for minor hair care as part of their makeup routine. This program is very successful with the Alzheimer's resident, as it helps to maintain and increase independence in activities of daily living. This routine activity is simple and rewarding for the female resident.

Group #3—For Your Eyes Only
Beauty Spot would not be complete without eyeglass cleaning. Use special glass-cleaning soap in spray bottles if you can, or just use soap and water. Again, be prepared. Soft towels and cloths need to be on hand to dry the glasses. It is a wonderful activity for the lower cognitive resident as they are able to handle most of the skills of the cleaning on their own.

Summary

Beauty Spot can easily take up an entire morning. Setup is crucial for a successful program. Be ready for your group. This group can be very diversified in cognitive levels. It is wonderful to see residents of various cognitive abilities interact and help each other with something they truly love. Caring for yourself and how you look remains an important concern throughout life. If the meaning of appearance changes at all, it becomes more important.

> *Nora paces the floor all day and much of the night. She is a resident in the Alzheimer's unit. She moves constantly. But when Beauty Spot is offered, Nora is always first in line and is easily able to hold her hands flat and still. Much of the time, Nora wanders around aimlessly trying to find her daughter. She is unable to stay longer than a few minutes in a group setting. As soon as Beauty Spot begins, we ask Nora to soak her hand in special moisturizing soap and she totally relaxes. She is able to stay with one hand soaking for at least ten minutes, then graciously puts her other hand in for another ten minutes. When the activity services staff is ready to work with Nora, she is still sitting down, waiting for her manicure. During the manicure, Nora smiles and enjoys her one-on-one time with the staff. There's nothing quite like personal attention and human contact. We carry that knowledge into all our groups, even those for higher functioning residents.*

Sports Stuff

The name of this therapeutic group tells you what it is about. Sport Stuff is a male-oriented group with a foundation in sports. This group can accommodate a variety of cognitive levels, and has proven successful with a wide range of interests in sports.

Goal: Provide a positive environment for men to share their love and interest in sports.

Objectives:

- Establish relationship with men of similar interests;

- Provide a variety of topics on sports to share and discuss;

- Provide the opportunity for men to teach each other skills they have had for many years; and

- Help increase memory skills.

Group Content and Setup

The group begins by passing around any one of a variety of pieces of sports equipment. Try a baseball and glove, a football, a golf club, tennis racket or a basketball. Each week a new topic is covered when an item is passed around.

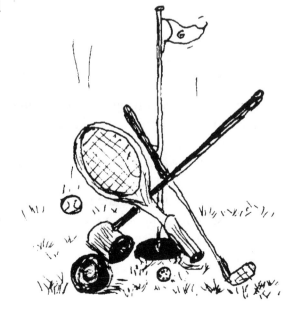

Once the equipment is passed around and experiences and interests are discussed, different topics are covered. Often the group can play a sports game. Try trash can basketball, tether ball, table hockey, or any other sports-related game. The game and your equipment do not have to be elaborate to be enjoyable. Magazine articles are read and discussed. *Sports Illustrated, The Sporting News* and *Sports Illustrated for Kids* are wonderful tools filled with interesting, current discussion topics.

Chapter Six

A male staff member best facilitates this group. It becomes a men's club, where only sports are discussed. Sports Stuff, you will find, is an enjoyable program for your sports enthusiasts. Your membership can include widely different cognitive levels. This means it's important to keep conversation centered around sports only. When the facilitator keeps discussion limited to one topic, the lower functioning residents find it easier to join in.

> *Ray was 89 and suffered from dementia. Ray was very active and continually walked around the facility. Despite all his energy, he couldn't communicate with anyone, not even his family. His family visited often, but they never really knew what to do when they came. They would sit with him, silent for the whole visit. No one would say anything. Ray would always attend Sports Stuff. Every time the group met, Ray would hold onto a baseball for the entire session. One day, the facilitator centered in on a discussion of baseball. The conversation was spirited. Everyone had a story to share about baseball, and everyone paid close attention to Ray. Then one member talked about the no-hitter he once threw in a minor league game. Ray began squeezing the ball and tightening his grasp. He curved his hand inward and formed a knuckle ball. All the members knew exactly what Ray was doing and congratulated him on excellent positioning of his fingers. He was enthralled. He continued to show the group various baseball holds and the group ended up going twenty minutes longer because of their interest in Ray's knowledge. This was a breakthrough for Ray and we made sure his family heard all about it.*
>
> *Following this meeting, his family brought in a baseball and they were able to pitch and catch the ball with him on every visit. Even at 89, Ray turned out to be a great ballplayer.*

Invite the Sports Stuff group on monthly outings. The group is perfect for ball games once a season. I also invite the group to pool halls and bowling alleys. This group ended up going out at night to see high-school basketball games in the community and even went to a horse jumping competition. Our Sports Stuff team became extremely close and usually sat together for special events and other happenings in the facility. The higher functioning residents would be responsible for reminding the lower functioning residents that the group was about to begin. They would even help transport those who needed help getting to the meetings.

Sit and Be Fit

Goals: Provide the opportunity to participate in physical activity.

Objectives:

- Help residents gain some strength and endurance; and

- Allow residents to meet others with similar physical fitness needs and interests.

Nothing new here. This is a simple exercise program. This is another group that will attract some residents, but not others, based on their history. This program or a similar one is already offered in most facilities. Here are a few more tools to help you run this program. As part of your screening, ask the facilitator these important questions:

- How do you know how far you can push each one of your residents in physical exercise?

- How do you warm-up and cool-down properly?

Make sure the facilitator has discussed the physical abilities of the residents with a nurse or physical therapist. Involve the physical and occupational therapy department, they are very educated in appropriate exercises for older adults. These departments will be flattered that the activity services department consider their involvement important in the lives of the resident. Most residents who enjoy physical activity are able to move in many different ways. Check with the nurse and go for it.

- How do you involve all your residents who have an interest in physical activity?

In your assessments, look at exercise as a part of their past lifestyle. All cognitive levels can participate in exercise. Keep in mind though, this is not the time to convert the nonathletic to being physically fit.

- How do you make it fun and worthwhile for the resident and for yourself?

Spend a half-hour in a set program of exercises accompanied by taped music. Choose your music carefully, always using familiar tunes. Create a tape that lasts a half-hour. The music should begin slowly. Ballads and instrumentals like "In the Mood" are a great way to begin. Frank Sinatra's tunes are also perfect exercise music. Pick up the pace with some quick tempo music. Songs by Glenn Miller are well-received. End your time with old favorites that everyone can sing-along in such as "Let Me Call You Sweetheart." The routine you establish has great therapeutic value. Your residents will remember your style and be more effective in increasing their physical activity and succeeding in the group.

Create a set of exercises that go from the top of the head to the tips of the toes. Keep the routine similar every time. Know and understand what the exercises you have chosen are doing for the residents, what part of the body is being helped. Explain to your residents the purpose of each exercise, and why they should work on keeping healthy. There are many exercise tapes, videos and classes that can help train your staff to run an effective exercise program for your specific clientele.

Use this time to educate on eating right. Explain what it means when you don't take time to exercise as often as you can. Give handy hints on how to exercise without working too hard on it. Can you walk to dinner every night?

Then, allow an additional twenty minutes to do hand massages for your residents. This is a very intimate and important time. Massage therapy is new to many residents. Approach this new program with consideration and honesty. Ask the residents if they would mind having their hands touched. Touching is very important to most residents.

Have lotion handy (donated by a cosmetics company) and rub the hand, starting at the tips of the fingers and ending at the wrist. Circle the fingers, and slowly move them, one finger at a time. Stretch out the fingers, one at a time. Use the "thumb crawling" technique on the palm and back of hand, slowly circling the wrist. Always talk to the residents and ask if they are feeling any pain or experiencing any discomfort. Move slowly, and talk to the residents as you provide the hand massage. This is a very simple technique. If you are interested in pursuing more hand massages, consult your physical or occupational therapist for training and ideas. This extra touch can allow your facilitators a chance to establish real rapport and connections with residents. Find the residents that this works with, and keep them for the second half of the group, but allow others to stay and socialize if they are interested.

Family Tea Time

Family Tea Time originated because I'd noticed that visiting a loved one in a nursing home is often difficult for family members. This group allows food and surroundings to play a major role in conversation and communication. The resident is in a host or hostess role which allows feelings of comfort and independence.

Family members are less stressed because their loved one is confident and in charge in a familiar setting. That simple familiar setting is tea, cookies, music and conversation. And it's not a sterile bed with a roommate and no place to sit down. It takes some preparation and planning, but Family Tea Time is a guaranteed success group.

Goal: To create a quality time with family members.

Objectives:

- Prepare a "normal" setting for residents to share with family members;

- Empower residents to help prepare a small social event; and

- Increase socialization with the family.

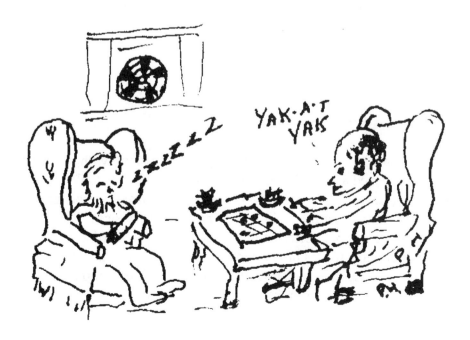

Chapter Six

This is a family-oriented group. This is designed specifically for the residents who continually yearn for and talk about their family. In Family Tea Time, we structure a social time with the family. The cognitive level of the resident has no bearing on the success of the program. This program allows the family to see the resident in a different setting than their usual visiting pattern.

Group Content and Setup

Send a written invitation to a family member. The invitation should read as follows:

> You and two friends are invited to share a social tea time with Resident's Name. On Date at Time in his/her room at Facility Name.
>
> Please respond to the Activity Services Department at Phone Number and Extension by Date, so appropriate plans may be made.

The tea is elegantly set up and held in the resident's room or a small lounge.

Supplies

- Teacups and saucers (ask staff and family members for the loan or donation of china cups, tablecloth and cloth napkins);

- A serving dish;

- Cutlery (including small spoons);

- Knife; and

- Food and drink to be served.

Set up a card table in a small lounge (or the resident's room) with tablecloth and the settings listed above. If the resident can help with the table setting, encourage him or her to do so. This allows the resident to take ownership of the event and gives him or her the feeling of being a host or hostess. The sense of ownership also comes with offering the resident a selection (from a predetermined menu) of items for his or her party. The menu can be as simple or as ornate as your food services department can manage. This sample menu might help when ordering from the dietary department.

Family Tea Party

For _____ Room #: _____

Date: _____

Location: _____

Number of Persons in Party: _____

Menu

Snack

Cookies
Crackers
Scones/Donuts
Crackers and Cheese
Muffins

Beverage

Coffee
Tea
Milk
Juice
Other: _____

Other Needs: _____
_____
_____
_____

Submitted by: _____ Date: _____

Day of the Party

The table and room are set up, and the family arrives for the tea party. Food and tea are served either by the resident or by the activity services staff. The resident (or family) chooses favorite music prior to the party. The activity services staff is available for cleanup or any other help. The party is usually a memorable one for resident and family. This type of activity, working with one family at a time, allows you to establish communications on a personal level with family members. This can make it easier to call upon them when you need their help in the future. This is a very special event for that family and should be offered once a year for each family. This is a small event and can be handled by one activity service staff member. It is successful when offered on Sunday, when there is a slow time before the facility's church service in the afternoon.

Chapter Six

Facility Chorus

Jane and Arnold had been active in bands and church choirs their whole life together. They had to move to our facility due to complications in Arnold's diabetes. Jane had experienced some memory loss, and couldn't control his medication correctly. The two of them stayed in their room most of the time. One day, the activity services staff suggested they come to choral practice. They did have some standards for quality, and guessed that the other residents would not be able to carry a tune. Finally, they agreed to come and watch a rehearsal. They were pleasantly surprised, and listened intently to all their favorite tunes. They hummed along with the chorus throughout the practice session, and came back to visit the very next rehearsal. After watching four practices, they decided to join the group. The choir's performance at a local mall, with their families present, will always be a highlight of their life at the facility.

Goal: To provide an opportunity for public performance for those who love to sing.

Objectives:

- Allow residents to meet with others who love to sing;

- Provide an environment conducive to all voices and levels of competency; and

- Provide an upbeat and harmonious group in which to socialize.

Group Content and Setup

This group is mainly for the high-functioning resident, mostly because of the demands placed on the chorus. The group rehearses every week and plans one performance every six weeks, either inside or outside the facility. Proper assessment for music interest and talent is imperative. The residents in this group become very close, and need the support of the other musicians in the group.

The props needed for this group are more cumbersome than many. A piano is needed, along with a pianist and a choir director. The best way to get this group off the ground is to find the "musical" staff in your facility. Comb the halls to find anyone interested in giving to the facility and knowledgeable about choirs and directing. If word is out that you are looking for musical talent, those who are interested will come forward. Staff members should also participate as singers or support people.

Your next step is to put a notice in neighborhood church bulletins. Ask for a choir director or pianist for one hour per week. This is often appealing to potential volunteers, because they know in advance that this is a limited commitment, and one that might prove rewarding. If notices in the church bulletins do not pull in the talent you need, try a volunteer bureau, or ask the entertainment editor of your local newspaper for help.

Encourage staff from all shifts to support the members. It gives the residents a feeling of importance and respect when staff members stop to congratulate them on their performances. The weekly rehearsal routine, the performances and participation of staff are all very therapeutic. It creates the most normal environment I have ever experienced in a nursing home. Your singers are transported in their minds onto a stage in front of an audience every time they practice. Anyone who has ever been part of a choir or chorus understands the emotions and connections allowed in such a group.

> *Amanda, a blind 94-year-old Alzheimer's resident, had sung professionally all her life. Amanda rarely spoke, but loved to sing. She lived to sing. The chorus director heard her singing one day and invited her to be part of the chorus. She never missed a practice. In the performances, Amanda loved to be up front, and would always hold the props we used, such as flags and hats. She loved being part of this group. I'll never forget one performance, though. The chorus was singing at the facility, in front of the families. Amanda was not feeling too well, and fell asleep right on stage early in the performance. When I woke her up after the show, she looked up at me and said, "I think I sang better than ever tonight."*

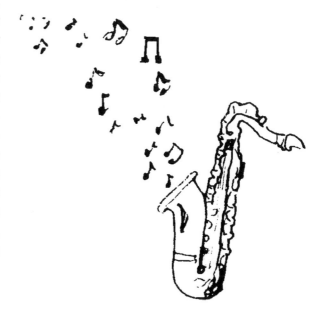

Sensory-Based and Alzheimer's Groups

7

These groups are designed to stimulate one or more of the five senses. Almost 90 percent of what we know is based on vision. The rest of what we know is derived from our other senses. However, residents with limited sight get most or all of their information about the world from smell, taste, touch and hearing. The sensory-based groups described in the following pages offer a variety of stimulation for each one of the senses. No matter what sensory limitations the resident has, these groups allow them to maintain or enhance their remaining senses. Perhaps fifteen to twenty percent of the residents in your facility may be visually impaired. Many of them will not be involved in diversionary groups. These sensory-based groups could help the visually impaired resident feel a sense of belonging that he or she might never again enjoy in any other way.

Groups discussed in this chapter—

- World of Nature

- A Touching Moment

- Read With Me

- A Sense of Smell

- Food and Such

- Music Appreciation

- Holiday Happenings

- Walk With Me

These sensory-based groups are also designed specifically for the lower cognitive or Alzheimer's resident, but membership does not have to be strictly limited to those residents. The higher functioning resident can be given specific roles and duties in these groups. Often the loss of a sense (for example, eyesight) will allow some higher functioning residents to feel more at ease with the lower functioning residents. The loss of one or more of the senses is the basis for the criteria for sensory-based groups. Most Alzheimer's residents will also fit the criteria of these groups.

Groups for Alzheimer's residents have been discussed throughout this book, but this chapter can be applied in total to their unique needs. It is imperative we provide quality programming for the Alzheimer's resident. Quality programming for Alzheimer's residents is difficult because of the variety of behavior patterns they exhibit. Whether it is difficult or not, quality programming must be provided, because it directly relates to quality of life. The first stage Alzheimer's resident is relatively independent in his or her ADLs. Once routines have been established, quality of life is the direct responsibility of activity services staff. We are responsible for the time the Alzheimer's resident is not involved in personal care routines.

The question then arises: How do you measure quality of life for the Alzheimer's resident? The answer includes points discussed in describing groups such as Sensations and Connections. These groups are oriented to the present, and intimacy is provided to attract the attention of the person with low cognitive abilities.

Alzheimer's is a disease that, in activity services, can only be dealt with by concentrating on the here and now. Success is measured in moments. If the resident does not exhibit aggressive or inappropriate behavior during a specific program, then the program for that resident is successful. It has been said that in many Alzheimer's residents, left-brain functions (e.g., language, reasoning, calculation) decrease and right-brain functions (e.g., feeling, intuition) increase. This has been taken into account in the design and development of these groups. They are not so much challenging to the mind, but instead are stimulating to the senses.

It is meaningful for activity services staff to understand the importance of the here and now. We cannot emphasize residents' ability to retain information or remember experiences. If this is difficult for professionals, it is particularly difficult for the families of the Alzheimer's resident to understand and practice. Many family members want their loved one returned to his or her former state. I often just tell them to remember how much their mother or father loved them, and to share that love now. Try to use the love that they received from their parent and redirect it, accept this "new" member of their family with love and support. Once the family can begin to accept their "new" member, they can begin to heal and continue their lives.

A good way to help family members understand Alzheimer's is to explain to them that the lexicon in the brain has been damaged. This analogy used to explain this concept has worked on many occasions. Explain that a lexicon is similar to a dictionary. If you tear out the pages of a dictionary, those words don't exist anymore. Similarly, an Alzheimer's resident can lose a definition, as well as the word connected to that definition, forever. This, simply stated, explains why certain words may have no meaning to their loved one, and why words might be used incorrectly, because the real word or its definition has been torn out of their dictionary.

Families play a big part in the sensory-based groups. It's very meaning-ful to have families involved and actively participating in these groups. The involvement you require from the family can be in various forms. Examples are provided as each group is discussed with tips on how to establish good family relationships.

One key difference between these groups and the other groups in this book is timing. Your ideal is a half-hour group, but if your group is reaching the residents and lasts ten minutes consider yourself successful. On an Alzheimer's unit, variety, flexibility and spontaneity are key components to a successful activity program. Connecting and intimacy are of prime significance.

Chapter Seven

World of Nature

World of Nature can be held throughout the year, but is most successful in the spring and the fall. We use nature soundtracks and items from nature to conduct this group.

Goal: To provide an opportunity to see, hear, feel, smell and touch elements of nature.

Objective:

- Provide an opportunity to identify items found in nature;

- Provide an opportunity to listen to sounds of nature; and

- Provide an opportunity to participate in environment surrounded by nature.

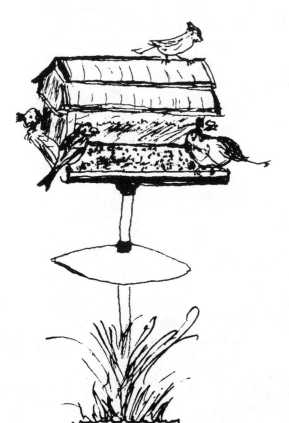

Group Content and Setup

The group is made up of any resident and his or her family that is interested in the outdoors. This could be open to all of your Alzheimer's residents. The residents and their families who have stated that they enjoy the outdoors, (e.g., fishing, walking, gardening) would be the first to invite. Limit the group to between eight and ten people and keep sessions to a half-hour in length.

Begin the group with a tape of bird calls or other nature sounds. You can also use waterfalls or ocean sounds, for example. Do not use relaxation tapes which sometimes include music or narration. The sounds need to be clear and easily identifiable. These tapes are available at your local library or at most bookstores. Before you begin to seat the residents, you should place nature-related items around the room. Your residents should be encouraged to walk around the room or sit near the objects that interest them the most. Have a variety of items spread around the room. Allow group members time to examine the items on the tables. Ask a resident to bring you specific items in the room. The more ambulatory residents will enjoy the fact that walking around the room is acceptable and even required as part of the group.

> *Fern constantly paced the hall near her room. She was unable to sit down, even for a meal. She was difficult to redirect when she had something on her mind. Music was always one of her favorite pastimes, but music sometimes sparked some painful memories for her. As we met for World of Nature one morning, Fern heard the sound of birds and walked into the room. She sat down immediately and rocked back and forth until calmness prevailed. She sat throughout an entire portion of the group, and then got up to leave. I recommended she come and examine some of the items I had on the tables, and she did. She stood by the leaf table and held each one individually. She commented and discussed each leaf for quite some time. She held a maple leaf to her heart and talked about the tree in her front yard that always dropped these leaves. Fern was placid for the entire group and every World of Nature group we had for the following three months. She found herself back at home in a peaceful, loving environment until she died.*

Objects that have proved to be successful:

- Leaves—all shapes and colors you can find;

- Pine cones and acorns;

- Rocks, stones, pebbles;

- Wildflowers, dandelions, weeds;

- Sticks and branches;

- Tree bark;

- Pictures of animals and birds found in the forest;

- Feathers; and

- A rabbit's foot or pelt.

Chapter Seven

It is recommended that all the leaves, flowers and weeds be pressed, then laminated and cut out. This allows them to keep their shape, and to be held without damage. The more items the group is able to handle and identify, the better. The group sits in a very small circle and shares the objects. If you are lucky enough to have a secure outdoor unit, you could use this time to walk around the facility with your residents and find items matching those they have in their hands.

All these items from nature are familiar to the residents, and much comfort comes from these items. Residents often have vivid memories that relate to these items. From World of Nature, I was able to develop a very active bird-watching group in the Alzheimer's unit at one facility. The unit was fortunate enough to have the participation of a Boy Scout working on his Eagle Badge. He developed a bird-watching environment, including a birdhouse and a bird feeder right outside the dining room. The residents were very involved with the birds. It became part of the routine in World of Nature to fill the bird feeder. The Eagle Scout provided us with laminated snapshots of the birds that could be spotted in the feeder and house. We placed the snapshots on a ring and hung the ring by the window of the dining room. Occasionally, an Alzheimer's resident would pick up the ring and flip through the pictures to find the bird that was eating seeds at that time.

The Eagle Scout came and spoke to the group on many occasions. The activity services staff had helped him prepare simple discussion topics, along with questions that were sure to hold the residents' interest. This bird sanctuary developed into an ongoing project. Part of the group painted bird houses and repaired feeders that had broken around the facility. The key to the success of this group is the same as the Boy Scout motto: "Be prepared."

Many family members were involved with this World of Nature group. They found items of interest as they walked around our grounds on their own. This involvement was easy for the families and was nonthreatening. It gave each family member some empowerment with their loved ones without too much commitment. An article was written for our monthly newsletter, describing the group and encouraging family participation. The response was overwhelming. Prior to the initiation of this group, even the facilitator had no idea how much nature was available in our area.

The items used for this group should be readily available for family visits. It is often difficult for a family member to visit a loved one with Alzheimer's. This box filled with "God's Garden" can be a catalyst for discussion and quality time spent with a loved one.

A Touching Moment

Touch can be such a forgotten sense in the nursing home. Physical touch is the essence of this group. Shaking hands as you welcome members into each meeting is a good way to start to this group. Thanking the members for coming as you close your meetings with a hug or handshake is also recommended. A Touching Moment is a group my residents have found to be most enjoyable. The response to it may very well prove outstanding in your facility, too.

Goal: To provide an avenue to use the sense of touch.

Objectives:

- Identify what you are touching or that you are touching something;

- Provide an opportunity to touch a variety of textures;

- Provide an opportunity to touch items they have not felt in a long time; and

- Provide an opportunity to use a sense little used in the nursing home.

Group Content and Setup

The group is positioned in a circle. The facilitator introduces everyone in the group, or asks those who can to introduce themselves. The key to this group is the creativity of the facilitator. The more inventive you can be, the more the residents will respond. Like most sensory based groups, A Touching Moment should not last more than a half-hour, and should not have more than eight or ten residents.

Part One
Begin with a large balloon, and fill it with a quantity of an item. Do not inflate the balloon. It is sometimes tricky to fill the balloon, but use your imagination. Often two or three activity services staff can work together on this. Two might hold the balloon open while the other fills it. Other times just using a funnel will work well. It can cause a mess but once the balloons are made, the hard part is done.

Chapter Seven

Recommended fillers:

- Coins (all types)
- Baking soda or flour
- Beads
- Beans
- Rice
- Nails, screws, bolts
- Confetti
- Buttons
- Peanuts, walnuts, pecans, pistachios
- Seeds or peach pits
- Pebbles, sand or gravel
- Spices
- Paper clips
- Marbles
- Cloves
- Magnetic letters or numbers
- Small figurines
- Cotton balls

The list is endless, but as you can see, the variety of shapes and textures you can place in your balloons is inspiring. The residents have great fun identifying, or trying to identify, the various "feels." This can be a difficult task at times, and can become annoying to the residents if it is done for too long, especially if the facilitator insists on residents identifying the items before moving on. The "feel" itself is the goal here. Just feeling something new and allowing the mind to explore new sensations is the goal of this group. Keep this going for as long as there is general interest.

Part Two

Part Two is very similar to a section of the group Storylines (found in chapter five). In Storylines, we place different items in a bag, and participants are asked to identify the items. In A Touching Moment, we use the same set of wooden items each time, placed in the bag with group members being asked to identify the items. The items are different shapes made solely of wood. The shapes are easy to identify and very distinct.

Prepare a set of items shaped as:

- heart
- triangle
- ring
- square
- pencil
- cylinder
- cube
- ruler
- fish
- circle
- mushroom

This portion of the group is fun, since it can create interaction between group members. Each member will help the other identify what he may be feeling inside the bag. The bag should be a dark color and should be made of soft velvet-like material. The dark color provides good contrast for the wood pieces and the soft feel is another added touch for memories. The identification of the items is not necessary for the success of the group. The feel of the items, the experience, is the reason we conduct this group.

Part Three

This is another "feeling" activity. This requires you to invest in some "pretend" fruit and vegetables available at a toy or craft store near you. The fruits and vegetables should be of comparable size to the fruits and vegetables found at your local grocery store. These items should be plastic and be as colorful and as realistic as you can find. The next step is to find real fruit and vegetables corresponding to the plastic ones. Ask the residents to identify what fruit or vegetable they are holding. Can they tell the difference between the real ones and the plastic ones? Can they smell the difference? What differences can they discuss? Each resident could hold a real and plastic fruit or vegetable and discuss their possession. The resident might try to eat the real (or even the plastic) food, so be prepared and keep a watchful eye. The fruits and vegetables we have found successful are bananas, onions, apples, pears, grapes, potatoes, green peppers, and tomatoes.

Summary

The group is divided into three parts, but does not necessarily require all three parts for each meeting. Allow the group members to direct the facilitator by their interest level as the meeting progresses. Perhaps only one part might be done in a single meeting. Again, be prepared. You will be glad to have additional ideas ready and waiting for the residents who are not responding to the initial ideas you thought were brilliant.

> *Laura, a bright, visually impaired 87-year-old resident, enjoyed the first part of this group. Her favorite containers were the ones with the coins inside. She would spend the group time holding on to the containers with the money and trying to identify the type of coins in the containers. Laura was usually a fussy woman who participated in few activities, but when A Touching Moment was scheduled, she would only fuss if she was forgotten or brought to the group late. She felt in charge of the group. Her cognitive status allowed her to lead the group in discussion on the various textures that the group was experiencing. Laura felt her presence was a necessary component for the group's success. The ultimate goal for this, and every group in this book, is to affect positive change in people's lives, one day at a time.*

This story gives an example of how higher functioning residents might be involved in any of these groups. You know your residents. Do not invite them if they might feel humiliated or insulted. Try a resident in a group one time and you will know if his or her participation is appropriate.

Chapter Seven

Read With Me

Goals: To help increase attention span.

Objectives:

- Provide an opportunity to hear favorite stories and poems; and

- Read easy-to-understand stories to increase use of attention span.

Group Content and Setup

Reading is a program found throughout nursing facilities. It is successful in room visits, using the Bible or a famous piece of literature. Read With Me is reading with a twist. This group is designed for the resident who has lost many of his or her senses except for his or her hearing. Hearing is necessary for participation in Read With Me. Depending on the material you present, the group might also be called Poetry Corner. This group has worked with a variety of cognitive levels. It is found that the residents with lower cognitive levels do not respond, or can even fall asleep in a group when the facilitator is not loud enough for them to hear. A portable microphone and amplifier is valuable in a program such as this. It is helpful for the facilitator to read slowly and with feeling and emotion. Read With Me often becomes a favorite for the residents who are visually impaired. Work at offering reading that is both educational and interesting to your listeners. Your visually impaired residents feel connected with the world when the world talks to them.

This is a very different group than Today's News (discussed in chapter five), because there is no discussion. The pieces read by the facilitator are not discussed or reviewed. The stories are feel good stories with happy endings. I recommend funny short stories rather than jokes. The poems are not deep or controversial, but easy to understand and light in tone. The stories can be from magazines or books. The size of the group is crucial. Keep it between six and eight. Seat the group in a semicircle and have the facilitator sit in the center of the circle for all to hear and see as he or she reads. An overattended group setting can prevent members from hearing the stories effectively. If you are fortunate to have a small tie-on microphone, use it. Never read for more than 30 minutes to avoid losing the group's interest The groups might be established on the basis of interest or cognitive level. You decide. Be creative and invite retired teachers to volunteer to read to the residents.

Humor can be a vital component to this group. Laughter is often missing in the nursing home environment. Stop for a moment and think about the last time a resident laughed out loud. This is a wonderfully contagious sound and is a highly recommended form of medicine. What makes people laugh? What makes you laugh? Try different stories, look for ideas. Ask staff members, "Have you seen Ellen laugh? What made her laugh?" These questions, posed to families or staff, are helpful in building your repertoire for Read With Me.

> *The most successful Read With Me Program I ever had was in Florida with a group of six Alzheimer's residents. I read the book* The Greatest Story Ever Told *in its entirety. This book is over 200 pages long. It took 50 weeks to complete. It is a story of Jesus written in everyday language. When I opened the book on the sixth or seventh group session, Curt said, "Is this the Jesus story?" On the twentieth week, Diane said, "Can we bless this book?" The same six residents stayed with the book from beginning to end. It brought me such comfort to see the peace this book brought each of those residents. When I closed the book and said, "The End," A. J. said, "Read it again!"*

Chapter Seven

A Sense of Smell

Olfactory activities in long-term care are on the increase. Activity service professionals have found that different smells provoke calmness and relaxation with the Alzheimer's resident. This finding is confirmed by many relaxation manuals and techniques used all over the world. Smell stimulates the senses and calms the mind. Most smells evoke positive memories. Positive memories provide a sense of self-worth which promotes contentment.

Smells such as chocolate chip cookies, bread or apple pie provide warm memories of home and family. Smells like those of flowers, pine trees and burning leaves evoke past environments and occasions. Even foul odors evoke memories, thoughts and discussion and increase stimulation to meet your objective.

Goal: To provide an avenue to use the sense of smell.

Objectives:

- Provide a variety of smells to provoke memory;

- Increase use of the senses;

- Provide a learning environment free of stress; and

- Offer opportunities for success.

This group is designed specifically for Alzheimer's residents or the resident who responds to smells. The sense of smell seems to intensify as one gets older. In fact, it seems to be more intense due to the decline of other senses. If this is true for some of your residents, this will be a very effective group. Smell can be a significant memory trigger. If a scent is part of one's past associations, it can be retained when other basics of life are forgotten.

Group Content and Setup

This is a relaxing, reflective group. It is a time where smells bring memories and thoughts back to the resident who has few other senses. Ideally this group is comprised of eight to ten residents and should last no more than a half-hour. In preparation for the group, collect as many film canisters as you can. Place a request in the facility newsletter and ask for families to donate small containers.

As the basis for our group experience, various fragrances are placed in these canisters. Close the canisters and put three small holes in the top. You need holes so the fragrance gets out without your residents getting into the contents. Place the same scent in eight to ten containers. Hand them out to all the residents in attendance, and ask questions such as these:

- What do you smell?

- What do you use this for?

- Is it used in the kitchen?

- Can you eat it?

- What are you thinking of when you smell this?

- Does the smell remind you of something or someone?

- Close your eyes and tell me where you have smelled that smell before?

- Close your eyes and tell me who was with you when you last smelled this?

The group can succeed with no questions as well. Provide the same smell for each resident and simply sit back. Allow the residents to say or "not say" whatever they please. Words can be meaningless during some groups.

Try things like onions, baby powder, lemons, spices, paint, chocolate, cinnamon, wild berries, vanilla, eucalyptus, raisins, basil, wild flowers, aloe, apple juice, tomatoes, gum, garlic, peaches, fresh bread, cookies, pies, cranberries, apples, pears, bananas, apricots, perfume, cologne or aftershave, shampoo, coconuts, and/or olive oil. When using a liquid to produce the smell, make sure a cotton ball is placed in the canister. To seal to canister, use transparent tape around the outside of the cap. This seals in the odor and keeps everything in the canister.

Avoid using relaxation tapes or massage during this group. These are excellent techniques but can take away from the purpose and goal of your group.

Allow the smells to bring on conversation and discussions. Often, oriented residents passing by will smell the incense or candles from the room and stop by. They will participate and end up contributing wonderful stories and anecdotes. This group, in some cases, is the only group that can reach certain residents.

Chapter Seven

Food and Such

Cooking and baking have always been successful with the residents because of their past experience in the kitchen. Many homemakers have years of experience accumulated in the kitchen. Food allows residents to succeed in an environment anchored in their past. The kitchen, its smells, and its familiarity are a comfort zone for the residents.

Cooking for the activity service staff must be taken seriously. The equipment, tools and supplies must be handled and accounted for by the staff. Alzheimer's residents have shown surprising recall of the purpose of the kitchen utensils. They seem to be able to handle the equipment, but one should be cautious, and *never* leave the residents alone during this group.

Goal: To provide an avenue to promote cooking and baking.

Objective:

- Touch, smell, see, and taste common foods;

- Provide a success-based environment that is familiar and comfortable;

- Use utensils and items residents have used in their past; and

- Cook and bake popular foods.

Group Content and Setup

This therapeutic group works well with a variety of residents with sensory deprivations. One resident may be visually impaired, another may be hearing impaired. Together they can work to accomplish some small, yet rewarding tasks. Food and Such meets weekly. The group I worked with prepared a dessert that was shared with the rest of the facility, or with the residents' wing of the building that same evening. The evening program is therefore easy to plan, as it revolves around serving and eating the afternoon baking delicacy that the group created. Our most popular project has been Friendship Bread (one of my employees brought the starter and recipe from home). You are certain to find many recipes by asking staff, visiting the library or searching the Internet. Sourdough bread starters are widely available at health food stores also. The Amish Friendship Bread project, once it is underway, is one that never stops. Each day the residents get involved with the work and

Amish Friendship Bread Starter

Dissolve 1 package active, dry yeast in ½ cup warm water (110–115°F) in a deep glass or plastic container. Add 2 more cups warm water, 2 cups sifted sugar and 1 tablespoon sugar. Beat until smooth. Cover with loose fitting cover or place in a resealable freezer bag. If you use the bag, be sure to open it and let the air escape once a day or it may burst. The starter requires 10 days for fermentation.

Amish Friendship Bread

Do not refrigerate. If air gets into the bag, gently squeeze it out.

Day 1: Squeeze the bag of starter
Days 2–5: Squeeze the bag
Day 6: Add 1 cup flour, 1 cup sugar, and 1 cup milk (or water) to the bag; squeeze bag to mix ingredients together. (This is optional, but it creates one more bag to give away.)
Days 7–9: Squeeze the bag
Day 10: Combine in a large nonmetal bowl:
the starter batter
1 cup flour
1 cup sugar
1 cup milk
Mix with a wooden spoon or spatula.
Pour four 1-cup starters into one-gallon resealable freezer bags.
Give three starters away and keep one for yourself.

This step refreshes the starter. Starter should be used within ten days.

Add to remaining batter:

1 cup	oil (or ¼ cup oil an ¾ cup applesauce)
2 cups	flour
1 cup	sugar
½ cup	milk
1 tsp	vanilla
½ tsp	baking soda
3 large	eggs
1 large box	vanilla pudding
1½ tsp	baking powder
2 tsp	cinnamon
½ tsp	salt

Pour into two large loaf pans that have been well-greased and sprinkled with cinnamon sugar. Sprinkle top with cinnamon sugar and bake at 325°F for one hour.

coordination of the project. It is a wonderful idea to have your residents serve their Friendship Bread as part of Family Night.

Make a Difference Day is sponsored every year by the USA Weekend Magazine. *It is a day when individuals and groups help out their community. The residents of our Alzheimer's unit wanted to do something for their community. They loved all the volunteers coming to visit them, and they wanted to make a contribution. Our opportunity appeared when we found a group home for the blind whose residents loved home cooking.*

Our Alzheimer's unit was known for its cooking and baking. This group could cook. It was their favorite thing to do. The baking and cooking programs were highly successful at holding participants' interest. Most residents stayed through any cooking program and helped out as much as they could. No matter what was being prepared, all the residents shared in the organization and production. Both the men and the women shared equally in the joy of cooking.

The group home for the blind was invited to enjoy a gourmet meal made from scratch by the residents on the Alzheimer's unit.

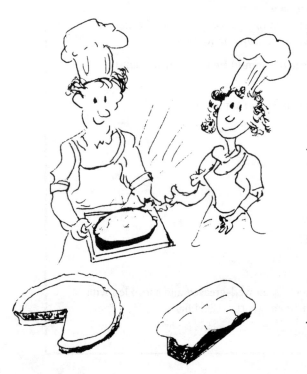

They were thrilled at the prospect of having a meal catered for them on this special day. Our plan was set in motion. The residents chose the meal. Family members donated all the ingredients for the meal. Our menu included tossed salad, ham, twice-baked potatoes, green bean casserole and rolls, with Dutch apple pie and ice cream for dessert.

Baking and cooking was on the calendar every day the week before the event. The family members were asked to volunteer some recipes and time to help out with the various courses. It became a family affair. Our volunteers were fascinated by the level of interest of the residents and their abilities in the kitchen. Make a Difference Day arrived, and cooking and baking began early in the morning with all the volunteers assigned specific foods and ingredients. The residents were also placed into groups, working on the things they enjoyed doing most. The meal was completed by 3:30 p.m., brought to the group home, and set up by 4:30 p.m.

Three activity services people, three volunteers and three residents were responsible for delivering the meal and presenting it. The group home members sat anxiously as the table was set and food placed in front of them. A volunteer pianist from the facility entertained while the guests awaited their dinner. The dinner was presented and our residents, staff and volunteers sat interspersed with the residents of the group home. It was a phenomenal evening and everyone had a wonderful time. This day indeed made a difference, and received national mention in the Sunday paper, but I couldn't tell you which group got the most out of it, our residents or those we cooked for.

Music Appreciation

Music appreciation is more of a listening opportunity than Music in Motion (found in chapter six). This group is specifically aimed at the Alzheimer's resident. The philosophy for groups with Alzheimer's is:

1. **Keep a flexible time frame.** Success can be equally attained in a ten-minute group as well as a 30-minute group. Let the group decide on its length for the session.

2. **Groups are not result driven.** The outcome for any of these groups is not important.

3. **Present specific, focused programs.** As in music appreciation, for as long as you have the attention of your group members, keep the program focused. Do not bring in a variety of music. Choose *one* type of music for each session.

Goal: To provide an avenue to use the sense of hearing.

Objective:

- Hear familiar sounds and instruments; and

- Provide a calm environment to listen to music.

Music groups are, without a doubt, the most commonly presented therapy in activity services. It is easy to use music as a form of therapy. It is also the most response-provoking therapy available in a nursing home. Music is often a key to communication. The music groups discussed in this book simply give you another view of a much discussed topic.

Group Content and Setup

Music Appreciation relates directly to listening to music with some concentration, and picking up information about the music itself. Music Appreciation is a very effective program for Alzheimer's residents. They are able to listen to music if it is the only sound in a room and there are no other distractions. Music provided for this group can vary as widely as the residents who are part of the group. We have used content ranging from different eras of classical music every week to just the works of a single composer. It helps considerably if the facilitator enjoys music and understands classical music and popular music from bygone eras, and knows the variety of music available.

Open each session by playing the music the residents know and love. Play tapes of the famous artists and encourage your residents to listen carefully. Work with popular music for ten to fifteen minutes. Then devote the second half of your session, if the residents are still engaged, to different musical arrangements. From jazz to chamber music, use variety to create an opportunity to reach your most unreachable resident. The liner notes on tapes and CDs, or books from the library will give you all you need to know to lead discussions, if necessary.

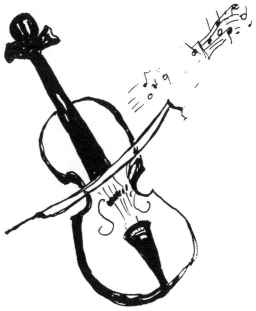

Chapter Seven

Holiday Happenings and Seasonal Celebrations

Greta was an 88-year-old woman with Alzheimer's disease. She was German, and spoke English with a very thick accent. Greta's family discussed her life story with the activity services staff. We noted that Greta loved the holidays, especially Thanksgiving. She had spent hours in the kitchen and prepared a ten-course meal for her large family each year. That was part of her legend. Every Thanksgiving, her family would get together and discuss their memories of their matriarch preparing and serving the meal. The activity services staff asked for the recipes and the traditions that Greta used year after year. We decided to re-create her legend in our own way. Holiday Happenings for that month was based on Greta's recipes and stories, and they were plentiful. Pictures of the meals and favorite prayers were discussed during the group. Even with all this personal history paraded before her, Greta's comments were few to the group. Then, one week before Thanksgiving, the group was memorizing the prayer Greta's family said before the meal. Suddenly Greta connected. She said, "Where are my children? They all need to be here and listen to this." A special, meaningful moment was shared. Greta had her most lucid moment in a long time, and we all learned from her family's traditions.

Goal: To use themes to arouse memories and emotions.

Objectives:

- Provide an opportunity to reminisce about a certain holiday;

- Provide reminders of special times in residents lives;

- Afford residents time to recall past events;

- Learn and share different traditions and customs; and

- Enjoy the company of people who share similar holidays.

Working with the holidays is a simple way to combine arts, crafts, music, current events, games and reminiscing all at once. Designing your activities around a theme makes programming straightforward and easy to facilitate. Planning can be done in advance for the entire year without any difficulty. Once you have designed a theme for a given holiday, keep all of your information in a single box. In subsequent years, all the information you have on file will still be valuable. Here are the seasonal and holiday themes I have used in the past:

1. New Year's
2. Martin Luther King Jr. Day
3. Valentine's Day
4. Spring
5. Easter
6. Memorial Day
7. Fourth of July
8. Summer Vacation
9. Fall
10. School Days
11. Halloween
12. Thanksgiving
13. Hanukkah (if appropriate)
14. Christmas

Group Content and Setup

The concept is simple, yet often it is not done in a meaningful way. Prepare your Holiday Happenings program to last for four weeks. That way you will have four programs that last between a half-hour and an hour. Separate each program into three to four parts with each section lasting about fifteen minutes. Again, if one part of your program is extremely well-received, be flexible and go with it. Enjoy what your group is enjoying, and don't be so strict as to create an unyielding schedule.

There are two ways to proceed with this group. As one option, you can prepare a multiweek program with different activities for each of the four meetings. Here's an example using Memorial Day, lasting four weeks:

Week One—The History
This can be your craft week. Prepare table decorations for the holiday with flags and patriotic emblems as the centerpiece. Choose two or three U.S. Presidents who were veterans of the service, and tell their life stories. Use trivia with military and patriotic themes.

Week Two—The World Wars
Play music from these time periods. Display reproductions of famous newspaper headlines. Talk about food, clothes and fads from the World Wars, using pictures and articles to stimulate discussion.

Week Three—Personal Notes

Discuss how your residents have celebrated this day in the past. Use a map of the United States and refer to it as you discuss where your residents grew up and lived their lives. Again, play period music from the world wars, and show documentaries on Memorial Day or the wars (available on video at most local libraries).

Week Four—The Celebration

Prepare the food together that you will serve at your observance. Discuss why Memorial Day is an important day. Invite children to come and hear stories about the wars from the residents. Learn and sing songs that are patriotic. Invite a color guard or military band to entertain.

Optionally, you can prepare a thematic program that is repeated for a few weeks leading up to, and on, the date of the holiday. As an example, here's how you might treat the theme School Days. Each group meeting follows a similar outline:

1. 10 minutes—Music and poetry including the word *school*;

2. 10 minutes—Show articles on the subject of school. (Use the materials from your Connections group, discussed in chapter four, including school supplies.) Using the supplies, like chalk and markers, flows nicely into the craft portion of this group.

3. 10 minutes—Make a simple craft each week (for example, consider paper apples with residents names on them for the windows, coloring or pencil drawings or finger paints, paint-by-number).

Walk With Me

Goal: To increase physical activity.

Objectives:

- Provide a safe and structured environment in which to walk;

- Provide a walking partner capable of protecting the resident; and

- Help decrease agitation by redirecting the resident.

Walk With Me is a physically active group I have used successfully with Alzheimer's residents. This group was part of a research project designed to modify the behavior of residents in the Alzheimer's unit in my facility. It is placed in the sensory-based groups because touching became a huge focus of this group.

It began by examining a pattern I had noticed. At the same time each day, our Alzheimer's unit seemed almost out of control. Every day from 3:00 p.m. to 4:00 p.m., almost every resident experienced a transition in their behavior. The residents would pace more than usual. They would become more verbally upset, as well as strike out during this time more than usual. This phenomenon has been noticed by others, and labeled *sundowning*. This label describes the time when Alzheimer's residents go through increased agitation and decreased abilities to handle situations.

There are a number of theories about the cause of sundowning. Researchers have stated that it is a time when residents might, out of force of habit, be changing gears. If they were a working person, they would be heading home at this time. If they were a homemaker, their children and husband would re-enter their life at this time of day. This time of day also corresponds with a change in shifts at most nursing facilities. Some theorize that this change increases uneasiness within the residents and causes them to be more unruly. It has also been said that late in the day (anywhere from 3:00 p.m. to 7:00 p.m.) climate and air pressure change, or the changes of patterns of light and shadow might lead to the changes in behavior we see in Alzheimer's residents.

None of these theories have been proven or confirmed. There are more questions than there are answers in this area. My colleagues and I took it upon ourselves to see if we could somehow offset the negative behavior we see at this time of day. This is why Walk With Me was created.

Chapter Seven

The first step was to have the families of the unit behind us for this research. With funding and cooperation from a charitable organization dedicated to Alzheimer's research, Trinity Foundation International, the following letter was sent out:

Date

Dear <u>Facility Name</u> Family Member,

Walk With Me is a new research project at <u>Facility Name</u>. As you know, research is of prime importance to the well-being of our residents at <u>Facility Name</u>. With the help of Trinity Foundation International, we are starting a new program designed to find ways to deal with behavior problems associated with Alzheimer's disease, more specifically "sundowning." Sundowning is a part of the disease process that occurs late in the afternoon. We are going to invite high-school students to walk and increase physical activity for the Alzheimer's residents every afternoon.

We would like your permission to invite <u>Resident's Name</u> to participate in "Walk With Me." It can only benefit your loved one to take part in this program. Accompanied by trained high-school students, participating residents will partake in regular exercise and we hope this will decrease their agitation during this time of day.

Please sign the permission slip below and return it to the facility. We would be pleased to have you come by between 3:00 and 4:00 p.m. any afternoon to meet the high-school students.

Kindest Regards,

<u>Signature</u>

The flyer on page 141 was developed to explain the project to potential volunteers and was included in the letter to the family member.

Walk With Me—What Is It All About?

Who?

We are inviting interested high-school volunteers to be part of a therapeutic research project sponsored by <u>Facility Name</u>. These carefully chosen volunteers will be working with the residents from the Alzheimer's unit.

Where? <u>Facility Name</u>

How much?

Time—We are asking that our volunteers commit to 30 hours of volunteer time beginning the first week of October and ending the last week of April. Our project runs about 30 weeks. We will ask volunteers for one hour at a time, once a week.

Why?

We are researching a phenomenon called "sundowning." During the late afternoon on any given day, an Alzheimer resident's agitation usually increases. The reason behind that increase in agitation is not known, but needs to be researched. We would like to see if we can distract them from their daily routine during this time with the company of a lively, young person.

We are looking for a change in the pattern of behavior. This is where *you* come in. We are going to promote physical fitness and go walking. The volunteers will walk around the facility (or outside if the weather permits) with the resident.

There will be a one-hour orientation in your school and a one-hour orientation at the facility. This time will be used to train the volunteer working with the Alzheimer's resident. A staff member from <u>Facility Name</u> will monitor the first hour with the resident.

When?

The Volunteer's Commitment (*Your* Commitment)
One hour per week, between 3:00 p.m. and 4:00 p.m., Sunday through Thursday.

Chapter Seven

A letter was then sent to several local high schools. Following the letter, the activity services director met with the guidance counselor or principal of the selected schools. The meetings were friendly and advice-oriented. The activity services director went with an open mind and an eagerness to learn from school administrators. Each school had different interests in the project. One school stated that the scholarship was unnecessary. They felt that participants' motivation should come from within. Another school told us that if we hand-selected the students, they would automatically feel a sense of ownership and empowerment. A third school described their volunteer requirements, so we fit our research and our program to their needs.

Once a relationship and commitment was set up with the schools, two one-hour orientation programs were established. One hour included a short documentary video and discussion at the schools, and the second hour included a tour of the facility and some time on the Alzheimer's unit. This time on the unit proved to be valuable. Students stayed in a group with the facilitator and simply observed the various behaviors of the residents. Time was set aside for discussion following the tour of the unit. This turned out to be a very beneficial time that allowed the students to talk about their fears, anxieties and misgivings.

Once the volunteers were matched with an Alzheimer's resident, they would walk together for one hour per day. There were 38 volunteers signed up with ten residents in the research project. The walking took place around the facility, and the residents became enamored with the students. After two weeks, the residents were waiting at the door for their new walking partners. This program received much positive media coverage and was extremely well-received by the residents and their families.

The research took a backseat to the day-to-day results we were witnessing with the residents and the young people. They established bonds no one ever dreamed possible. The walking continued until the end of April when the student's volunteer hours were completed or they were beginning their summer jobs. A number of students continued throughout the summer. This project will continue next September without thoughts of discontinuing this group in the future.

More details and a program guide for "Walk With Me" can be obtained at http://www.trinityusa.org or by writing to: info@trinityusa.org (e-mail) or Trinity Foundation International, PO Box 402, West Chester, Ohio 45071.

Drew and Sally were a match made in heaven. Drew, a tall, blond-haired young man, resembled Sally's husband. Her husband would visit in the morning and Drew would visit Wednesday afternoons.

Drew would walk with Sally throughout the facility. She never stayed far from Drew. At any time during their walk, one could see Drew holding hands and discussing his life with Sally. He never expected a response and never received one, but that didn't stop him from sharing his life with her. It wouldn't surprise us to see Drew wipe Sally's nose or arrange her hair. He had no qualms about "caring" for Sally. Drew fulfilled his volunteer commitment, but continues to visit her until this day.

Other Settings for Therapeutic Groups

8

Retirement Communities and Assisted-Living Communities

All the therapeutic groups outlined in this book can be used in the nursing home setting, but not all of them carry over into other environments. When reviewing therapeutic groups for subacute or retirement communities, careful scrutiny of the residents is mandatory for effective programming. The key to successful programs is complete and accurate assessments. As mentioned previously, nursing home populations have changed. Similarly, retirement communities have changed in recent years. The retirement community is no longer made up of first generation retirees. The first generation retiree is defined as being in the first ten years after retirement, ages 65–75 years old. First generation retirees who once would have considered a retirement community are staying in their homes longer. They are using their resources to support themselves there. Despite the advantages of home mainte-nance, housekeeping and standby nursing care, the first gen-eration retiree no longer looks at the retirement community for rest and relaxation.

The second generation, ages 75–84 years old, is now the generation looking for the retirement community living style. This has many implications. A major factor is the change in-volved in marketing the retirement community to older, more frail adults. The amenities included in the retirement package are more nursing-oriented and care-oriented than ever. We are now dealing with a form of assisted living offered as a retire-ment community living.

Chapter Eight

There is a concern with activity services in today's retirement community. The discipline has not changed with the new population of retirement communities. This is a significant problem. Often, the activity director is inexperienced, untrained or both. He or she "likes people," and thinks being with older people is fun and easy. With a more demanding population in the retirement community, it is more important than ever to hire activity services professionals with a background in therapy and knowledge of the older adult.

The activity services department in the retirement community often neglects to use a comprehensive assessment. It is not required, and is often viewed as nonessential to activity services. At this time, there are very few communities which do assessments on residents upon admission. This is a serious oversight for the department and for the administration to make. Often the marketing department feels like it is too nursing home–like to ask these past lifestyle questions in a formal way. I have found that the family and resident enjoy answering these questions, and it helps in planning a diversionary calendar as well as therapeutic groups.

If the activity services staff do not attempt a meaningful assessment of retirement community residents, then many needs will be left unmet. An assessment does not guarantee the residents will have all their needs met, but it will allow the department to fill as many needs as possible. It is advisable to have a simpler, shorter assessment form, which still inquires about a variety of activities and interests. The assessment's goal is to help focus the resident into a set of appropriate group activities. (See Appendix C for an activity analysis that has proven to be successful.)

Moving into a retirement setting is a traumatic experience. It can be comparable to moving into a nursing home. The resident is leaving behind many of personal possessions and moving into a smaller living space. New residents are eager to be part of a group of people who are experiencing the same emotions and feelings as they are.

Therapeutic groups are chosen for different reasons in the retirement community. The lower cognitive functioning groups would not be beneficial in this setting without modification. Many interest-based and high-functioning groups will work perfectly. Of course, you must use your judgment, and tailor the details of the group to your membership. Certain approaches recommended in the nursing home group could seem condescending or patronizing in the retirement community. Use your professional estimation of your membership as you tailor each group. Once appropriate assessments are completed, virtually any group in this book can be useful, and adapted to suit the cognitive levels and interests of the residents in the retirement and assisted-living facility.

Here is a list of the groups to start your program in the assisted-living and retirement community living:

- Welcome Club
- Show of Hands
- Reflections
- Pen Pals
- A Special Friend

- Puppy Pals
- Beauty Spot
- Memory Lane
- Sit and Be Fit

- Let's Talk Dirt
- Storylines
- Faith, Hope and Charity
- Family Tea Hour

Abe was in a nursing home for five weeks of rehabilitation. He was recovering from a series of serious strokes that left him blind in one eye. The therapeutic groups in which he was involved in the nursing home were A Show of Hands and Sports Stuff. Abe was a brilliant retired artist. He was very successful in these two therapeutic groups even though he was much more talented than his peers. In A Show of Hands, he enjoyed the projects and helping other residents with art projects that he could do simply and with much success. After his five weeks he was ready to move to an assisted-living facility. He needed help with his medications and a few of his ADLs, and the retirement community he was going to was designed to meet those needs. He moved, and although his daughter visited on a regular basis, he had no interest in participating in the programs being offered at the ALF. He did not enjoy going to parties. This is a classic case of the resident who needs therapeutic groups adapted to the retirement community. It was fortunate that the two facilities were connected and the activity services staff were aware of his involvement in therapeutic groups. The activity services staff added A Show of Hands to their calendar the week Abe arrived and it became a popular group at the retirement community as well as an artistic release for Abe.

Assisted-living facilities (ALFs) are fast becoming the "helping home" of the older adult. ALFs are springing up in communities all over the United States, and chains are forming in all parts of the country. One of the appeals of the ALF to owners and developers is the limited amount of state and federal regulation on their operation. Nursing home owners are finding that ALFs are more appealing to the older adults of the 1990s and beyond. They provide comforts such as weekly housekeeping, lawn care and snow removal, home maintenance, medication reminders and the convenience of someone else making breakfast, lunch and dinner. ALFs are able to provide a homelike environment where residents can receive limited medical assistance (perhaps from a home healthcare agency associated with the ALF).

Owners and operators can provide these comforts to private pay residents, and avoid altogether the regular monitoring and interference from unresponsive government agencies. Bankers and investors recognize a significant opportunity to receive good returns on their investments. Expect the trend toward assisted living to continue. It has built up significant momentum.

Many older adults are home alone, with no social contact outside of their television and irregular family visits. Families know this, and sometimes feel guilty about it. One reason families suggest an older adult relocate into an ALF is for socialization purposes. This is why a comprehensive, well-thought-out activity program plays such a significant role in the promotion and marketing of ALFs. Families can provide an environment in which their loved ones are not alone, and can have company any time, day or night. A well-designed activities program, presented to prospects, can become a major selling point.

The retirement community resident is more independent than the resident in an ALF. ALFs differ only in the amount of service offered. ALFs provide a wide variety of help with ADLs. In both environments, activity program design needs thought and careful consideration of the population and their interests. An assessment is included in this book for activity directors to use (see Appendix C). The assessment is simple and informal, but fulfills the most important purpose for the department. This allows you to welcome a resident effectively and make him or her feel you are there for him or her. This is the first connection you have with the resident. Keep in mind that you are not trying to fix the resident, or work on any particular problem as you might in the nursing environment. You simply want to know enough about your residents to help them form networks and friendships in their new home.

For new arrivals, I suggest a welcome sign appropriate for the facility, and then a visit from one of the activity services staff. Use that visit to conduct an assessment. Do not use the word "assessment" in your conversation, since it does sound a bit clinical. Properly conducted, though, your first visit is a good way of forming a relationship. This is an essential bonding time with a new resident. The resident is almost always willing and able to talk about himself or herself, and enjoys doing so. This assessment can be a starting point for a resident that is having a difficult time adjusting. Using this tool does not make your facility too nursing home-like. It helps to establish a relationship and establish programs that make sense for the resident in your facility.

Groups are then formed after the assessments are gathered and analyzed. Complete the group assessment procedure and find out what groups should be offered to your facility. Try the groups. If they are not a smashing success, you have learned something. If they do work well, so much is gained. Creating healthy relationships through these groups in a retirement community and in an ALF is the main purpose of providing these opportunities.

Subacute Care

The term subacute immediately describes a certain type of individual. This is not to say that one can stereotype the patient or resident in a subacute unit. The individuals are from a variety of backgrounds and leisure activities. They have different physical problems. There is one generalization one can make on a subacute unit: There is a potential for rehabilitation, and the majority of patients will be moving on either to a full-time placement in a nursing home or return home with in-home healthcare.

The physical, occupational and speech therapy departments play a vital role in rehabilitating the subacute care resident. Your activity services department should work in conjunction with the physical therapy, occupational therapy and speech therapy departments. Set your groups to revolve around their schedules. Work with the therapy departments to create programs that will benefit residents who are in need of speech, occupational and physical therapy treatment. The therapeutic groups can support the goals of the therapy departments and still attain great success at meeting the therapeutic recreation goals of the subacute resident. Making this cross-disciplinary connection can be very helpful to the activity services department. It allows you to focus on what really matters to the people you serve. What really matters is that they get better and get home. An activities component to traditional therapy can make a difference.

The most important area of concentration is the assessment for the subacute resident. Use your assessment to place the resident in a group as quickly as possible if he or she feels able to participate in a group. Make it clear to the resident that any and all therapy will help him or her regain strength, endurance, flexibility, and allow him or her to get home as quickly as possible. The resident may have many arguments against participation, but if the therapy department is behind the activity services staff and supports the therapeutic groups, your groups will be successful.

The groups that work best for subacute residents are simply small versions of any therapeutic group discussed. You can probably spare enough staff to place two to four residents in a small number of groups. The groups are based on the cognitive levels of the residents. Count on your subacute residents being involved for between 10 and 60 days. Know that these residents are working hours every day to increase their stamina and get back home. Do not try to schedule them in more than one or two groups a week. Know their problems, and help in their areas of weakness by providing groups tailored for their participation.

Group Therapy in a Nursing Home— What Is the Purpose?

The concept of group therapy for the older adult is relatively new. Its biggest obstacle is that the elderly population has not been exposed to this technique and often is not willing to communicate its feelings openly in a group. Often older adults are unable to find the trust necessary to communicate their feelings. This sharing of feelings is not something with which today's residents have grown up. The baby boomers will be too verbal when they hit their 80s, but the residents in nursing homes today were not brought up sharing intimate feelings and emotions. Despite this generational limitation, there is value in psychological therapy for seniors that often benefits them and their family members in profound ways.

Group therapy is usually associated closely with the social services department. The department will recommend a resident be seen by a psychologist for help with a particular issue. The most obvious problem that is faced by the psychotherapist is the fact that some residents have various forms of dementia. These can be very hard to diagnose. Are the residents behaving this way due to the fact that they are not adapting to their new surroundings or because they are in the first stages of Alzheimer's disease? You must have a truly *good* professional working with your facility in this capacity; someone who can readily identify where he or she can do the most good for residents and their families, and someone who will apply their energies effectively to the meaningful problems they face.

It is important to discuss this group therapy process in addition to the therapeutic groups in this book because of one factor: Therapeutic groups use the same concept of goals and objectives that are central to group therapy. This is how both disciplines evaluate their success with residents. If there is no consulting psychologist in your facility, I would recommend that you establish a relationship with one. Find out if there is a good therapist in the community or at another nursing home. A consulting psychologist is necessary to help you deal properly with intense and profound individual problems that are either too involved or need objective interference to help the resident solve his or her problem. Psychotherapists help people adapt to their new living situation. They offer support for residents who are dying. They guide residents and family in resolving differences. They are able to be objective when staff and residents differ on hygiene and living issues.

The social services department is able to handle the day-to-day problems (i.e., putting out fires), but the therapist examines these issues and problems in a more involved way. They look at problems, and assist residents in dealing with their present situation.

Facilitating communication is a key goal to most group therapy meetings. A good therapist will enable all the residents in the group to accept each other unconditionally. This enables them to accept help and wisdom from each other. Many times, residents can be critical of each other. The group therapy model helps the criticism to be redirected and focused by the group therapist. Unhampered communication within the group helps establish relationships. It is important in a nursing facility and it does work.

The most profound example is one I personally experienced. I think this experience explains the need for the expertise provided by this important group of professionals. The activity services department had scheduled a lunch outing at a nearby restaurant, and one of the coordinators had a great idea to invite the couples in the facility to partake as a group. Four couples attended the event.

Allen and Rosemary were a favorite couple, because five years back they married at our facility. Allen had told all of us that steak and eggs was his meal of choice and for this outing, he would indulge. The lunch began unusually gleefully with Allen and Bob exchanging war stories that became "fish" stories. Laughing and trading anecdotes was definitely the norm of the day. Allen did not make it home. He choked immediately following his last bite. Even though the staff acted and reacted professionally and expediently, Allen died before he got to the hospital.

This was, simply put, the most traumatic event I have ever experienced in almost twenty years in the long-term care business. There were five activity services staff present along with the eight residents. After Allen's death, going back to work was, for each of my staff members, nearly impossible. There was no escaping the fear, guilt and hopelessness we felt that day. Immediately upon my return to the facility, I called our consulting psychologist. The next day was his visiting day. I called to tell him that a number of his group members were probably going to need extra counseling. The psychologist suggested that all the residents and activity services staff that were present at the luncheon attend the group therapy meeting. We all attended, but with trepidation.

The group began with the members sharing their sorrow for the loss of Allen. They shared with Rosemary how much everyone enjoyed his company. Bob expressed his happiness that he had finally found a fellow Marine as a friend. The group members were able to speak when they felt like it, but the psychologist directed the group to fully understand the depth of what happened to each person in attendance. Each aspect of the event was discussed and every activity services staff member was able to partake at the level he or she felt necessary for his or her own personal healing process.

The residents' comments were powerful. Betsy expressed her desire to die in a place away from this facility, "A normal place, a place where people laugh and share their lives with one another, I want to die like Allen." Bob said, "I can't really understand the intensity of this event because the activity services staff acted so quickly and professionally and removed all of us from the area that we really didn't know what happened." Margaret said that she felt like she was surrounded by her guardian angel because the activity services staff protected and loved her so much.

The comments were extremely meaningful to all the activity services staff. This sharing experience would never have taken place if group therapy was not a vital and integral part of the facility. The psychologist knew the importance of meeting and dealing with this situation immediately. This was the first and most important step to the residents' and staff members' healing process. It was traumatic, and tough to deal with, but our psychologist handled all our needs with wisdom and kindness. Without that group and its excellent facilitation, I, for one, would never have realized what a profound impact the residents' reactions and comments were to accepting life and its unusually cruel possibilities.

Restorative/Activity Groups

Is there a way to turn your activities program into a revenue base for your facility? If there is a way to do that, then it could lift your department's credibility and status significantly. Reimbursements are a key to survival for the privately owned facility. Revenue generators get more attention and more resources, as well as more respect. Well, it turns out to be quite possible to bring in revenue with a quality therapeutic activities program, and the author is working toward that goal with a new concept called Activity/Restorative Therapy (ART). This is a new and exciting program still in its infancy. This portion of the book will just whet your appetite, because the details are still being worked out in a pilot program as of this writing. More will be available regarding reimbursements and the ART program concept in future publications.

Activity/Restorative Therapy still needs to be developed further, but merits mentioning. This concept is related to the restorative therapy programs currently being run in most facilities. This takes the concept one step further, and allows activity services to be just as involved as restorative aides in helping maintain a resident's abilities. The restorative aides are mostly involved with the clinical aspects of physical therapy. The ART aide would focus on motion, physical therapy and development of skills needed for ADLs. The idea is simple. Activity services can perform restorative services and generate revenue for the facility. Of course, regulations and requirements will vary from state to state. Make sure your program is eligible for reimbursement.

Here is just one program idea that allows you to conduct therapeutic activity groups, and entitle your facility to apply for state reimbursement as you go. Set up a program in which one of your staff, an ART aide, will facilitate exercise therapy programs to restorative patients. Active range of motion is a needed therapy. The ART aide is not just exercising one person. He or she is presenting an exercise program to a group of four residents. The group meets every weekday for a half-hour to an hour to work on movement and activity. The state regulations will state a minimum number of minutes per resident per day, and a maximum number of people in a group. Design your program to ensure all your state's requirements are met by your ART program.

Exercise is varied and simple and follows a set pattern week after week. Working with the punchball and balloons are part of the everyday group. Parachutes, Nerf balls, balloons filled with various items (see A Touching Moment in chapter seven) and music fill much of the time. This program is offered to the same restorative-eligible residents every day.

Chapter Eight

If you find it difficult to sell the concept of therapeutic activities to your administrator, mention that your ultimate goal is to use the programs as a revenue source. Our pilot program has shown that a good therapeutic activities program is a natural springboard into the ART concept.

Tools of the Trade

9

The activity services department is so often left in the dust when it comes to being heard and respected in most facilities. This department must promote its programs, be visible to the public, and be central to the daily operation of the facility. If the facility sponsors a seminar, fund-raiser or other event it should be under the auspices of the activity services department. Make sure that everyone from marketing to maintenance knows your plans and your accomplishments.

Do not sit back and permit the other departments to overlook your accomplishments or take credit for them. Do not base your professional reputation on making the best punch or playing the most bingo. Dedicate your department to the betterment of the facility and the residents that live there. Develop a department that is known for its creativity and uniqueness. Your staff must be prepared every day to be leaders in the facility. Be tenacious. Empower the staff to see the facility as their own and become a part of something big. Being leaders in the facility is a demanding responsibility. The responsibility never stops. Whether you have one staff member working on a Sunday afternoon or the entire staff at a large function on a Tuesday evening, your staff must be do-ers, and learn to be leaders.

When your department is represented in care conferences, you and your staff cannot simply report the number of events Rosemary has attended. You must question why she is not speaking with other residents during the event. Along with reporting the number of residents attending programs, you must also analyze and communicate what is happening during programs and events. Take a proactive approach to solving residents' problems. Most activity services departments use participation sheets to record the activities in which the resident is attending. These participation records should become individualized and reflect your plan of care for the individual resident. (See Appendix C for a sample participation sheet.)

Note that a column is added to check the activities addressed on the care plan. For example: You are promoting socialization for Elizabeth, and your assessment tells you she loves music. You will invite her to participate in all special music programs and invite her to become a member of Music Appreciation. On Elizabeth's care plan you have addressed that she will attend two music programs per month and Music Appreciation four times a month. You will immediately place a mark on the first column to signify the activity you are trying to promote and the second column with the number of times she should participate in that chosen activity. The information will be transferred every month until it is reviewed at her next care conference. At that time you will know if the care plans need to be modified or remain constant for another three months.

There is also space at the bottom of the participation record to write the name of the therapeutic group and (in the same column) the number of times you expect the resident to attend this therapeutic group. This helps focus the participation records to reflect the person you are trying to represent.

Some state governments require that you keep track of the activities the residents are attending. The state surveyors will review your participation records after they have researched the Minimum Data Set (MDS). Use your MDS to create your participation records. The general activity preferences found in the MDS should be clearly outlined in your participation record. In the example provided, the MDS activities are indicated with asterisks. If you have checked one of the MDS activities, the activity service staff must concentrate on inviting that resident to attend that activity.

In creating your participation sheet, avoid adding programs that do not mean anything. Games represents all the bingo, horse racing and tick-tack-toe you can offer. This still ties in with the plan of care that states the resident has always attended weekly bingo games at the church. Use the participation records carefully. As activity services director, you must get in the habit of auditing your participation records on a bimonthly basis. If there are blank sheets, then two things can be happening: Either your staff is not recording the information efficiently or you are missing the boat with that resident. Either way, you must act on the information you find.

In an Alzheimer's unit, the activity services staff can lack vision when setting goals for residents. The participation records become even more vital on this unit. They can be individualized and detailed for each resident. Working on very specific areas for these residents is imperative for effective activity management. There is a line provided on the bottom of the page to add addenda for specific residents. If the resident is not able to stay in the group for longer than five minutes, this would be written on this line. In the box, a star can be placed whenever the resident stays longer than five minutes. Again, after three months of recording this detail, the care plan can be analyzed and changed if needed. Your care plans are written with the help of these participation records.

Remember that each group in this book has a goal and a purpose. It can be a simple goal of socialization, but for many residents that is a significant change in their life. For example, if Blanche is verbal and creative, but finds life in the nursing home unsatisfying, the activity services staff might invite her to participate in Storylines (see chapter five). One of the objectives for this group is to promote socialization. There are other objectives, but that is the one that suits Blanche best. When you assign Blanche to a therapeutic group, her care plan is already partially written. The goals of the group would be the basis of her care plan with modifications to suit her needs. The problem would be her potential risk for self-isolation if she is not involved in any activities in the facility. Her beginning goal would be to attend Storylines once a week. This goal becomes easily measurable and can be followed closely on the participation records.

When it is time for the care conference, the goal can be examined and changed to suit what Blanche has done in the past three months. The activity services staff can see whether:

a. She has attended every one of the group meetings and enjoys them. Next step: Increase participation and add another group with more involvement such as One-On-One.

b. She is not attending at all. Next step: Change the goal to attendance at one Storylines per month, or choose another socialization group for her potential involvement.

c. She is attending, but has not decided whether she enjoys it. Next step: Maintain the goal and add interventions that involve the activity services staff visiting and reviewing the happenings in the Storylines group, and inviting group members to visit her.

Using this approach, care plans literally write themselves, because well-defined goals are the key to the therapeutic group concept.

Chapter Nine

This is where good computer software helps the activity services department improve its value to the facility. The software I use is a nonaccounting-based Windows package called the Facility Management Database (refer to http://www.sashacorp.com on the Internet). This software completely covers the needs of the activity services department like few other programs do. It can provide efficiency and cohesion in the process of programming, implementing and facilitating therapeutic groups effectively. It will also help you create care plans that are individualized and resident centered.

What the computer can do for the activity services department:

- Document and organize all therapeutic groups the department offers;

- Track the staff, day, time, and location of each group;

- Set up the goals and general notes needed to get the group off the ground; and

- Track date started and whether or not the group is active at this time.

As mentioned in other areas in this book, groups will be successful for various reasons. Such things as the season, the residents currently in your facil-

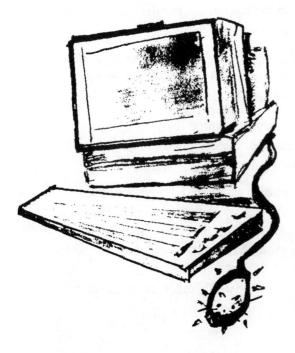

ity, and available staff will all be factors. These reasons and many more will lead you to start or end a group. The Facility Management Database tracks each activity group with an active/inactive flag. This enables you to track groups you have done in the past along with your current ones. This can serve as a reminder to bring successful ones back to the forefront. Dropping a group is not a sign of failure. The only way to succeed with therapeutic groups is to incorporate change into your program offerings. Change in the activity services department is good. It keeps staff and residents involved and interested.

Setting up groups is your first step. Include all of the groups you are interested in and make sure you have staff allocated for each group. Do not set up a group without a staff member in mind. The idea of the group is not nearly as important as its implementation. Each group should include the main goal you are trying to achieve with the group. Do not be afraid to change the major goal from the ones written here. You know your residents well. You can create what works best for them. With the Facility Management Database, complete the section of the database dealing with group master records (see Appendix D for sample screens and reports from the database).

You will need resident information for your department to use this database effectively. Once your current residents are entered into the database, assign your residents to the groups you want them involved in. In addition to tracking membership, the system allows you to determine specific goals for each resident within the group you have chosen. There are also tools in the database to help track residents based on their former lifestyles and occupations. Along with cognitive level, these are two good indicators of what your residents have in common with each other, and where you are likely to be successful in encouraging socialization.

The Facility Management Database allows the activity services department to record information on every resident in the facility, and find any person that might have fallen through the cracks—residents who for various reasons are not included in programs. The activity services staff think they have programs for all of their residents. With complete and current information, you can make better decisions about group assignments, or lack thereof. You can often make decisions about group assignments by selecting from residents who are not active in groups or diversionary programs. Their therapeutic groups are chosen by placing them in a low/high interest-based group that works for each of them.

You would be surprised how easily your group assignments fall into place. Once you've assessed all your residents, you will find a group that works for each of them. It is very important to ensure that every resident is participating as much as he or she is able. You can simply create a group called "diversionary" for residents who are not interested in small groups and are happy with bingo, morning coffees and special events. Remember to establish a room-visit group for the residents who are room-bound. This permits visits by activity services staff and other residents. Try to get the room-bound resident involved with a group such as One-On-One, or Faith, Hope and Charity. Every resident is then accounted for and participating, and that is the ultimate goal of any activity services department.

159

Good computer software offers you operating efficiency. When residents in your database are given a move-out date, they are automatically pulled from all your activities schedules, along with 200 other available reports. This saves you the time of rewriting dozens of records a day, and gives you more time to design and implement services.

The Internet

Computers are the department's eyes to the world. So often the activity services department runs its department on past experiences and ideas. That is not acceptable when useful information is at your fingertips. This information runs the gamut, touching every aspect of what activity services do. If you are interested in current events for therapeutic groups such as Today's News or Read With Me, *USA Today* and dozens of newspapers are available on-line. Searching for weather trends for A World of Nature? Government agencies and news media can give you anything you need. The computer is your dictionary and your encyclopedia. It provides answers for questions brought up in groups, and it provides questions to pose to your groups.

The Internet, more specifically the portion called the World Wide Web (www), can be your idea provider. There are newsgroups and reference sources on the Web for every group discussed in this book. If you need simple ideas for crafts, use search engines like Webcrawler, Yahoo! or Alta Vista to explore arts and crafts on the Web. For detailed information on a specific resident's interests or disabilities, the Internet brings a massive library to your desktop. If you have an artist with dyslexia, or right-handed paralysis, search for: *creative AND art AND therapies* in one of the search engines, and ask an expert. If you need to create material for your Trivia Time because someone in the group has stumped you, look for: *trivia AND entertainment*. If a group member in your Movie Mania is arguing about what kind of dog Toto was, then look up *Wizard of Oz*.

This is just a taste of what the Web can offer in the way of helpful hints for your department. There is no end to the resources available on the Web. Knowing what is available, and how to find it is only half the equation. One must have the equipment and support resources needed to make searches on the Web possible. There are definite necessities that the activity services director must insist upon. These include a personal computer, a high-speed modem, a separate phone line for the computer and an account with an on-line service or an Internet service provider. These basic informational tools are becoming very commonplace. The system, the Internet access and the software to organize your department is not too much to ask for. All of it is a worthwhile investment for your facility.

Making It Happen 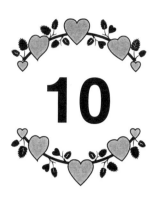 10

The concept of therapeutic groups is based on resident assessments and individualizing programs for the resident. The key to effective and successful therapeutic groups, beyond all the concepts and planning, is only one thing: *the perfect activity services department.*

This is not as difficult as it seems to be to attain. Everywhere I have ever worked I have been able to achieve this simple yet mandatory requirement: Make groups work. Whether you are lucky enough to have eight activity services staff persons or work alone, there are techniques that produce quality management and effective groups.

1. **Plan your groups according to the interests of your activity services staff.** If you like gardening but none of your staff does, assigning a staff member to Let's Talk Dirt guarantees failure. Do not offer Radio Daze if no one on your staff is older than 24 and none of them have ever heard of Fibber McGee and Molly.

2. **Allow your staff to choose groups that interest them.** Do not assume you know what group they want to facilitate. This provides the sense of ownership you are looking for with each group provided in your facility.

3. **Review, evaluate and organize your groups with staff participation.** What would work in this facility? What would never work? Go through the assessment provided in this book with your staff, analyzing your resources before you analyze your residents (see Appendix C).

163

Eliminate groups you don't see working in your facility for some reason. For example, Memory Lane will not work if you do not have a bus available to you on an ongoing basis. Use this form as a guideline to help decide which therapeutic groups you will offer. Now you are ready to proceed with the resident's personal assessment.

4. **Accept *all* of the relevant changes that your staff suggest, even if you don't agree with the details.** Allow them to succeed or fail on their own terms. The groups they run must be *their* groups. Empowerment plays a significant role in the success of a group.

5. **Prepare the groups with your staff.** Take time to help them prepare all the basics for each group. As an example, you can prepare the boxes together for Connections, making sure all the boxes are clearly marked. Take an active role in accumulating the items needed for all the different groups.

6. **Watch your groups closely.** Offer to facilitate each group first and allow your staff to watch. Observe the group until the facilitator tells you directly that they are no longer in need of your help.

7. **Keep asking about the group.** Listen attentively to the facilitator's comments about the residents involved. The activity services director learns much about the residents from their staff. They are your eyes and ears. Be there for them after every group. Listen to their stories.

8. **Analyze your groups quarterly.** Involve your staff with the evaluation. Ask "Why is it working?" or "Why is it not working?" Are the appropriate residents in each group? Are there others who should be attending? Evaluate the group for at least three months. This allows failures and successes to be apparent, and opinions to be based on facts rather than prejudgments. If the group does not work, discuss why, and make sure the activity services staff facilitating the group does not take it as a personal failure.

9. **Constant evaluation of your groups is needed.** You must be willing to change with the residents. Is the group going stale? Is

the group following the program? Is there a switch in the interest in the group? A prime example would be a group like Connections; if not properly directed, it can become a reminiscing group. This is not the goal of Connections. That is not to say that reminiscing with the residents is bad, but it is inappropriate for this group. Look at situations constantly, and help your staff examine whether or not a reminiscing group would be more successful in this case. Create *new* groups. Use the ideas in this book as a springboard to creativity. Adapt them to your facility, your climate and your environment. Be creative and innovative together.

10. **Don't be afraid to make a mistake—The one-on-one interaction a resident receives in a group will not be wasted.** Evaluate and acknowledge all your staff's success stories as well as their failures. Be prepared for errors in evaluation, and changes in your residents, too. Be prepared to move the residents to the group that best suits them. Moving a resident or canceling a group is not a failure. Your time is never wasted if you are *learning* as you go.

11. **Be enthusiastic about your therapeutic groups.** If you are excited about your groups, the staff and your residents will be too. You must support your groups at all times. When people criticize the exclusion of residents from a specific group, be kind and explain the goals and objectives of that specific group. Say something like, "Gertie will be going to her own therapeutic group later today. We chose Connections for Gertie because of her interest in school."

12. **Praise often and *mean* it.**

These points are vital for the success of the groups. Working with your staff closely as you put groups into play, following these twelve points closely, will create a *perfect* activity services staff. These techniques will create bonds and build teamwork and camaraderie. It took many years of teamwork to develop and refine these groups. These groups were tested and perfected and discussed with all my staff members on a continuous basis.

Working together following these guidelines is all designed to better the life of your residents. What could be more rewarding? What more stimulation does your department need to work perfectly? Keep in mind (unless you work alone): You are *not* your department. Share this wealth of information, and share the power to change things with your staff.

I know what you are thinking: "This is too time-consuming."

An investment is required to make all of this happen. Setting up a program of therapeutic groups is time-consuming. This is where I will prove to you that, with good time management skills, you can keep things going and still plan and implement successful therapeutic groups. The following example is set up for a facility of 100 residents and two activity staff persons, the director and an assistant, although staff/resident ratios vary greatly from state to state and from facility to facility.

Fact: Out of 100 residents, 25 are very involved and satisfied with diversionary activities the facility is presently offering.

- Out of the remaining 75, ten are room/bed-bound and will not or cannot come out of their room.

- The remaining 65 residents are not involved on a profound level with anything in their environment. Reasons for this have been previously discussed.

Fact: Staff members are paid for 40 work hours per week.

- Out of those 40 hours, eight are consumed by writing the daily activities on the board, chatting with residents and just hanging around.

- Out of the remaining 32 hours, about ten are spent on program preparation, care conferences, assessments, care planning and progress notes.

- Out of the remaining 22 hours, eight are given over to diversionary activities, and another two hours are spent transporting residents to and from those activities.

- After this routine, there are 12 hours remaining in the week, and you are left with these hours to facilitate your therapeutic groups. This only accounts for one staff member's time.

No staff member should facilitate more than two therapeutic groups per day. As previously mentioned, each group should last no more than a half-hour. This takes up five hours per week. Remember to allow two hours of staff time to transport residents to and from therapeutic groups.

The remaining five hours allow your staff to properly prepare and organize for the therapeutic groups that are offered, and give you time to follow up with staff to ensure they are successful.

> *Fact: From my experience, I have stated that the ideal number of residents in a group is between five and ten. Each group and its members will be unique, so each group must be analyzed separately. For discussion purposes, let's say that we will offer eight different groups in our sample environment. We have 65 residents in need of services. This works out to about eight residents per group, with each of the 65 attending only one group a week.*

This is a realistic assessment of the way we spend our time, and how we could spend it more effectively. We now have our 40 hours broken down to the minute. You will not have any unproductive time. You will be busy. You will not have a moment to spare. But my point is simple: It can be done. With the resources you now have, and with some thought and caring, you can create a meaningful program for every level of cognitive ability and interest.

Do not get hung up on the numbers. You may have a more demanding schedule. You may have more staff per resident. You may get nurse's aides to do all your transportation to groups. You may have to take on other duties yourself. Every facility is different, but no matter what your environment, everything I am recommending is possible. The details in my example are simply an eye opener, to show you how much more you can accomplish in your department. Try not to feel overwhelmed about adding more to your calendar. Look at this as an investment. It will produce rewards, and help you to connect with the residents who need you the most.

> *With our example, we have created enough time for ten groups, so why not go ahead and offer that many? As long as every resident who needs services is getting them, it's good for your residents to participate in more than one group.*

Chapter Ten

Preparation

Before you endeavor to begin your therapeutic groups make sure of a few things:

1. **Discuss the importance and the purpose of your program with the executive director, administrator, and all the decision makers in your facility.** Have the programs you will be offering documented and offer a written proposal to the administrator. The administrator needs to be behind this new and creative activity program. It is going to take time to educate the entire facility. The administrator must back you 100 percent.

2. **Discuss the importance of this new endeavor in your care conferences.** Be sure all the disciplines know that they are part of the success of your therapeutic groups. Let them know the kind of results you expect to achieve. Make clear that you will share the credit with them once your goals are reached.

3. **Evaluate your residents.** Know who you are dealing with. If you are new to a facility, take three months before initiating any groups. Find out who lives there. Determine the level of family involvement. Read the assessments already written on each resident. Find out whether they are complete, in the sense of answering the questions you need answered. Find out what has worked in the past. Do not "reinvent the wheel." Are there groups in place that are successful? Apply a simple twist to make them meaningful therapeutic groups.

4. **Evaluate your working environment.** Know your staff and how much they get involved with residents and with program planning. Know what kind of activity services staff you have to work with. Do you have to change a mind-set with the administration concerning daily bingo games?

5. **Be flexible.** If a group is put in place and its goals are not being achieved, look at it from several angles. If the group is successful in terms of providing enjoyment to its members, then perhaps you can change the goals. Examine your goals as much as you examine your results.

6. **Do not be disappointed.** Members of some groups, especially Name Game and Sensations, will not always respond as you would desire. Make sure your goals and objectives are attainable. If you see that there is no way the residents can attain these goals, you have two choices: Either change the goals or move the residents to more appropriate groups. There is nothing written in stone—these programs are for your residents.

7. **Teach everyone in your department how to master the skills involved in running therapeutic groups.** No one should be indispensable with regards to facilitating these groups. Some of your staff will enjoy it more than others, and that is totally acceptable. Make sure everyone can run a group, and can do most of them from experience. All your staff should understand the importance of therapeutic groups to your department's reputation and credibility, and more importantly what they mean to the residents.

8. **Keep your groups on a schedule.** It is important to the residents once they begin to feel ownership of their groups that they know when and where the group will take place. Be consistent, and keep everyone informed.

9. **And most importantly, *be prepared.*** Do not begin your group without preparation, and all the supplies and props you need. If you are not educated, confident and prepared, you have failed your residents. If you meet all those standards, you cannot fail.

10. **Have Fun!**

Learn and create, share and love. You are the life of the facility and you are family for your residents. You know them better than anyone. Promise me this: When something good happens (and I know it will), think of me. Thanks for sharing my dream.

Supplemental Material for One-On-One

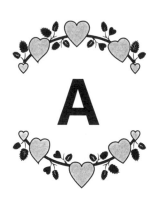

A

Appendix A

Visiting Schedule

Sunday	Monday	Tuesday	Wednesday	Thursday	Friday	Saturday

Please sign the day you visit

Supplemental Material for A Show of Hands

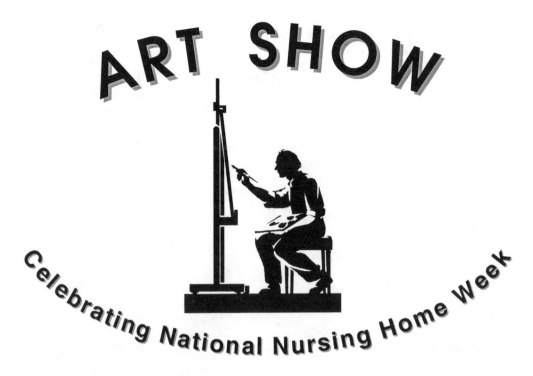

ART SHOW

Celebrating National Nursing Home Week

To feature entries on the theme:

"The Joy of Caring...Generations of Life"

Sponsored by _____

Original entries by Elementary and High-School Students

Entries must be submitted by _____

Public Exhibit on _____

Great Prizes to Schools and Individuals!

Entry Slip

Title of piece: _____

Name: _____

School: _____ Grade: _____

Age: _____

Media: _____

Certificate of Achievement

In recognition of your contribution to the
National Nursing Home Week Art Contest

Presented on this _____ day of _____

to _____

_____

Sponsored by

Administrator

Resident Assessments

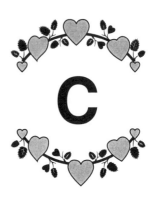

C

Appendix C

This assessment will help you select or reject groups for a resident. Ask each question on the right hand side of the form and put a checkmark (√) in the 'status' column of appropriate groups, and an 'X' next to the ones you eliminate. If you end up with both an 'X' and a check next to a group, eliminate that group for this resident.

Resident: _____ Date: _____ Room Number: _____

Group Name	Status	
1. Beauty Spot		IF THE RESIDENT:
2. Connections		
3. Facility Chorus		enjoys crafts, select 23
4. Faith, Hope and Charity		enjoys music, select 3, 12, 13
5. Family Tea Time		enjoys gardening, select 9
6. Food and Such		enjoys the outdoors, select 9, 35, 36
7. Holiday Happenings		enjoys movement, select 24
8. Hospitality Club		is new to the facility, select 34
9. Let's Talk Dirt		enjoys personal grooming, select 1
10. Light Touch		enjoys sports, select 28
11. Memory Lane		enjoys animals, select 17
12. Music Appreciation		IF THE RESIDENT IS LOW COGNITIVE:
13. Music in Motion		
14. Name Game		**eliminate** 4, 8, 11, 15, 16, 20, 27, 29, 30
15. One-On-One		
16. Pen Pals		and has no specific interests, select 2, 10, 21, 26, 32
17. Puppy Pals		and needs sensory stimulation, select 6, 22, 31, 36
18. Radio Daze/Movie Mania		and enjoys music, select 7, 12, 13, 18
19. Read With Me		and enjoys movement, select 10, 24, 33, 35
20. Reflections		and is verbal, select 2, 14, 18, 26, 32
21. Sensations		and loves to be around people, select 5, 7, 33
22. A Sense of Smell		and is room-bound, select 1, 5, 10, 17
23. A Show of Hands		IF THE RESIDENT IS HIGH COGNITIVE:
24. Sit and Be Fit		
25. A Special Friend		**eliminate** 2, 6, 7, 10, 14, 18, 19, 21, 22, 26, 31, 32, 35, 36
26. Spell and Tell		
27. Spelling Bee		and has no specific interests, select 20, 30
28. Sports Stuff		and enjoys people, select 4, 8, 15, 34
29. Storylines		and has excellent long-term memory, select 8, 11, 20, 27, 29, 30
30. Today's News		and religious, select 4
31. A Touching Moment		and room-bound, select 1, 4, 5, 8, 15, 16, 17, 25
32. Trivia Time		
33. Walk With Me		
34. Welcome Club		
35. The Work Group		
36. World of Nature		

Activity Analysis

Name: _____ Nickname: _____ Room: _____

Move-in date: _____ Date of Birth: _____

Interests

☐ Current Events ☐ Sports ☐ Socials ☐ Writing ☐ Exercise
☐ Restaurants ☐ Pets ☐ Cards ☐ Outdoors ☐ Eating
☐ Movies ☐ Parties ☐ Reading ☐ Bowling ☐ Travel
☐ Shopping ☐ TV ☐ Games ☐ Music ☐ Discussions
☐ Outings ☐ Crafts ☐ Children ☐ Spiritual ☐ Theatre
☐ Gardening ☐ Beauty ☐ Singing ☐ Birthdays ☐ Radio

Specific Interests/Other: _____

Past Involvements

Church _____ Home _____
Work _____ Friends _____
Community _____ Family _____

Preferences

☐ Individual ☐ Small Group
☐ One-on-one ☐ Large Group

What would you like to learn? _____

Is it easy for you to meet new people? _____

How do you feel about learning a new activity? _____

What did you do after you retired? _____

What did you do in your community for fun? _____

What is the most important thing for you to have in your new home? _____

What are you excited about in your new home? _____

Signature: _____ Date: _____

Resident Participation Record

Resident: _____ Date: _____

Activities	X	1	2	3	4	5	6	7	8	9	10	11	12	13	14	15	16	17	18	19	20	21	22	23	24	25	26	27	28	29	30	31
* Arts and Crafts																																
Beauty Spot																																
Bingo																																
* Cards																																
Discussion/News																																
* Exercise/Sports																																
* Games																																
* Gardening/Plants																																
* Helping Others																																
Meetings																																
Men's/Women's Club																																
Movies/Radio/TV																																
* Outings/Trips/Shopping																																
* Read/Write																																
* Religious/Spiritual																																
Room Visit																																
Self-Directed																																
* Sing-Along/Music																																
Special Event																																
Therapeutic Group																																
Walking/Wheeling Outdoors																																

O Observed R Refused
S Sleeping T Therapy
F Family √ Other
B Beauty Parlor * MDS Activity

Room: _____ Therapeutic Group: _____

Computer Software Sample Screens and Reports

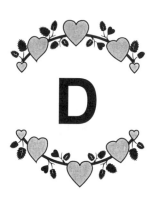

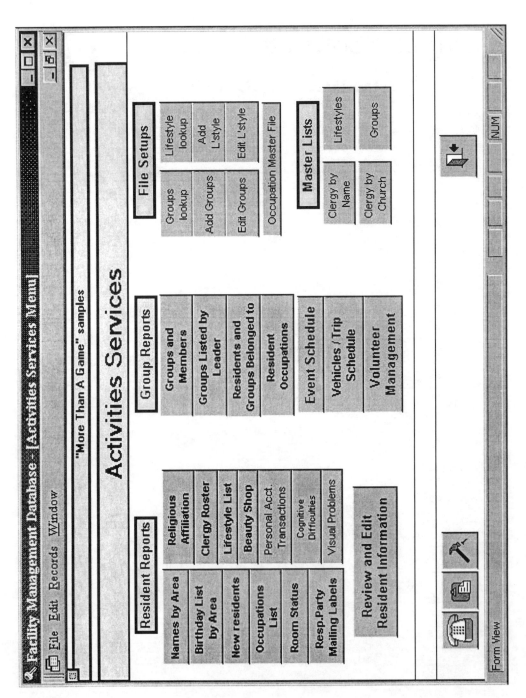

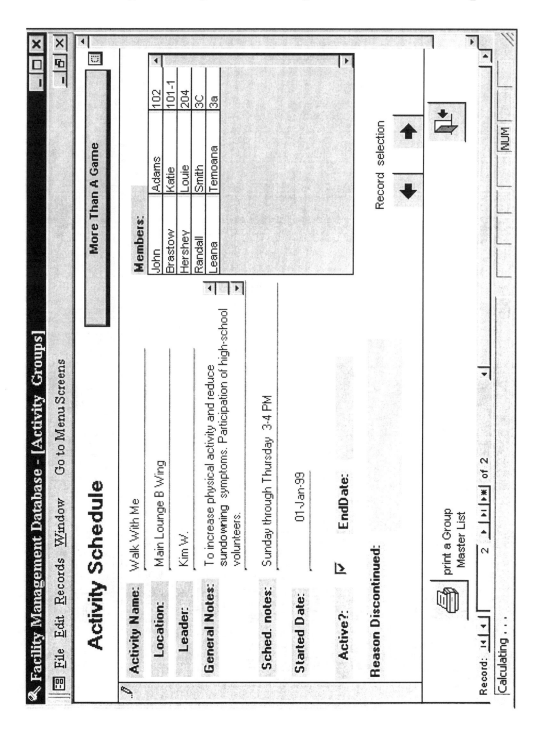

Appendix D

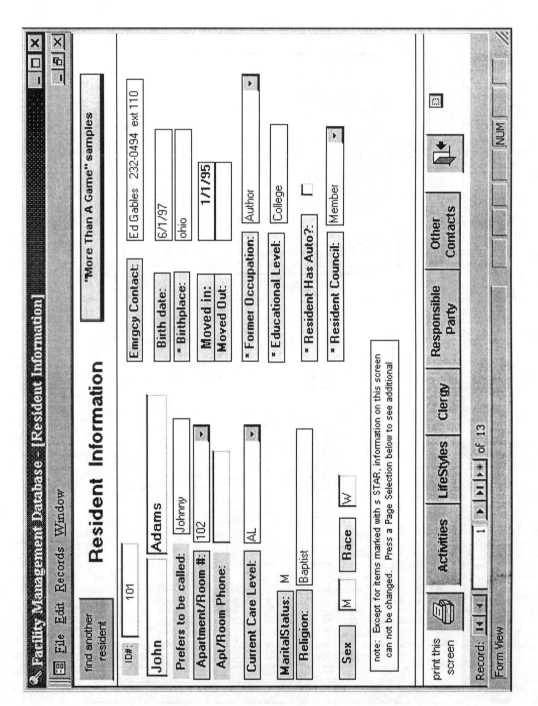

Facility Management Database - [Activity Group Membership]

File Edit Records Window

Activity Group Membership

"More Than A Game" samples

John | Adams

ActivityGroupName	Leader	Date Joined
A Touching Moment	Shelby	31-Dec-00
Goals To help increase use of sense of touch, particularly the left hand.		
Let's Talk Dirt	Kelly	31-Dec-00
Goals To increase use of left arm, improve strength and manual dexterity while gardening.		
Walk With Me	Kim W.	31-Dec-00
Goals Increase ability to redirect during each walking experience		

Add new info   Refresh display

Record: I◄ ◄ 1 ► ►I ►* of 3 (Filtered)

Form View   FLTR   NUM

Activity Groups by Leader

Leader	Group Name Members		Date Joined
Kelly	**Let's Talk Dirt**		
	John	Adams	31 Dec 00
	J. L.	Heist	31 Dec 00
	Shirley	Weise	31 Dec 00
Kim W.	**Walk With Me**		
	John	Adams	31 Dec 00
	Rose	Avenue	31 Dec 00
	Katie	Brastow	31 Dec 00
	J. J.	Hershey	31 Dec 00
	Ruth	House	31 Dec 00
	Mark	Markess	31 Dec 00
	Trixie	Skittles	31 Dec 00
	Randall	Smith	31 Dec 00
	Leana	Temoana	31 Dec 00
Linda	**Holiday Happenings**		
	J. J.	Hershey	31 Dec 00
	Ruth	House	31 Dec 00
	Mark	Markess	31 Dec 00
	Trixie	Skittles	31 Dec 00
	Randall	Smith	31 Dec 00
	Today's News		
	J. L.	Heist	31 Dec 00
	Zelma	Johnson	31 Dec 00
	Grace	Jones	31 Dec 00
	Leana	Temoana	31 Dec 00
	Shirley	Weise	31 Dec 00
Monica	**Reflections**		
	Zelma	Johnson	31 Dec 00
	Grace	Jones	31 Dec 00
	Leana	Temoana	31 Dec 00
Shelby	**A Touching Moment**		
	John	Adams	31 Dec 00
	Ruth	House	31 Dec 00
	Name Game		
	Katie	Brastow	31 Dec 00
	Mark	Markess	31 Dec 00

Activity Groups by Members

Group Members	Leader	Group Goal Individual Goal
A Touching Moment	Shelby	**To provide an avenue to use the sense of touch.**
John Adams		To help increase sense of touch, particularly in the left hand.
Ruth House		To increase dexterity of both hands.
Holiday Happenings	Linda	**To use themes to provoke memories and emotions.**
J. J. Hershey		To respond to one direct question asked during each group.
Ruth House		To identify each holiday correctly.
Mark Markess		To stay for the entire group (30 minutes) without asking to leave.
Trixie Skittles		To create one craft item each month.
Randall Smith		To recount one story of his past during each group.
Let's Talk Dirt	Kelly	**To provide residents with hands-on experience with dirt and gardening.**
John Adams		To increase use of left arm, improve strength and manual dexterity while gardening.
J. L. Heist		To participate in group 4x/month and help the other residents.
Shirley Weise		To maintain all potted plants in the facility weekly.
Name Game	Shelby	**To establish an opportunity to help identify the resident's name and the names of the other group members.**
Katie Brastow		To identify name during each group.
Mark Markess		To identify name during each group.
Today's News	Linda	**To provide a forum to discuss current events.**
J. L. Heist		To increase socialization 4x/month and discuss issues with other group members.
Zelma Johnson		To meet new friends and help adjustment to nursing home placement.
Grace Jones		To stay informed on current events of the day.
Leana Temoana		To stimulate long-term and short-term memory.
Shirley Weise		To increase leadership role in facility.
Walk With Me	Kim W.	**To increase physical activity.**
John Adams		To increase ability to redirect during each walking experience.
Rose Avenue		To follow all directions during group.
Katie Brastow		To maintain current walking skills.
J. J. Hershey		To respond to volunteer each day and call volunteer by name.
Ruth House		To maintain ability to walk independently.
Mark Markess		To stay focused on walking with volunteer and not wander off with staff.
Trixie Skittles		Increase walking to 5x/week.
Randall Smith		To stay focused and walk during group.
Leana Temoana		To help other residents by walking with them.

187

Group Summary Chart

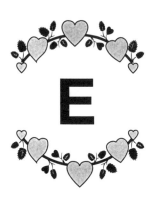

GROUP	Low Cognitive	High Cognitive	Intergenerational or Family-Based	Interest-Based
Beauty Spot			√	√
Connections	√			
Facility Chorus			√	√
Faith, Hope and Charity		√	√	
Family Tea Hour			√	√
Food and Such	√			
Holiday Happenings	√			
Hospitality Club		√		
Let's Talk Dirt				√
Light Touch	√			
Memory Lane		√		
Music Appreciation	√			
Music in Motion				√
Name Game	√			
One-On-One	√	√		
Pen Pals		√	√	
Puppy Pals			√	√
Radio Daze/Movie Mania	√			
Read With Me	√			
Reflections		√		
Sensations	√			
A Sense of Smell	√			
A Show of Hands				√
Sit and Be Fit				√
A Special Friend			√	
Spell and Tell	√			
Spelling Bee		√	√	
Sports Stuff				√
Storylines		√		
Today's News		√		
A Touching Moment	√			
Trivia Time	√			
Walk With Me	√		√	
Welcome Club				√
World of Nature	√		√	
The Work Group	√		√	

Other Books from Venture Publishing, Inc.

The A•B•Cs of Behavior Change: Skills for Working With Behavior Problems in Nursing Homes
   by Margaret D. Cohn, Michael A. Smyer and Ann L. Horgas
Activity Experiences and Programming Within Long-Term Care
   by Ted Tedrick and Elaine R. Green
The Activity Gourmet
   by Peggy Powers
Advanced Concepts for Geriatric Nursing Assistants
   by Carolyn A. McDonald
Adventure Education
   edited by John C. Miles and Simon Priest
*Aerobics of the Mind: Keeping the Mind Active in Aging—A New Perspective on Programming
   for Older Adults*
   by Marge Engleman
Assessment: The Cornerstone of Activity Programs
   by Ruth Perschbacher
*At-Risk Youth and Gangs—A Resource Manual for the Parks and Recreation Professional—
   Expanded and Updated*
   by The California Park and Recreation Society
Behavior Modification in Therapeutic Recreation: An Introductory Learning Manual
   by John Dattilo and William D. Murphy
Benefits of Leisure
   edited by B. L. Driver, Perry J. Brown and George L. Peterson
Benefits of Recreation Research Update
   by Judy M. Sefton and W. Kerry Mummery
Beyond Bingo: Innovative Programs for the New Senior
   by Sal Arrigo, Jr., Ann Lewis and Hank Mattimore
Both Gains and Gaps: Feminist Perspectives on Women's Leisure
   by Karla Henderson, M. Deborah Bialeschki, Susan M. Shaw and Valeria J. Freysinger
The Community Tourism Industry Imperative—The Necessity, The Opportunities, Its Potential
   by Uel Blank
Effective Management in Therapeutic Recreation Service
   by Gerald S. O'Morrow and Marcia Jean Carter
Evaluating Leisure Services: Making Enlightened Decisions
   by Karla A. Henderson with M. Deborah Bialeschki
The Evolution of Leisure: Historical and Philosophical Perspectives (Second Printing)
   by Thomas Goodale and Geoffrey Godbey
File o' Fun: A Recreation Planner for Games and Activities, Third Edition
   by Jane Harris Ericson and Diane Ruth Albright
The Game Finder—A Leader's Guide to Great Activities
   by Annette C. Moore
Getting People Involved in Life and Activities: Effective Motivating Techniques
   by Jeanne Adams
Great Special Events and Activities
   by Annie Morton, Angie Prosser and Sue Spangler
Inclusive Leisure Services: Responding to the Rights of People with Disabilities
   by John Dattilo
Internships in Recreation and Leisure Services: A Practical Guide for Students, Second Edition
   by Edward E. Seagle, Jr., Ralph W. Smith and Lola M. Dalton
Interpretation of Cultural and Natural Resources
   by Douglas M. Knudson, Ted T. Cable and Larry Beck

Other Books from Venture Publishing, Inc.

Other Books from Venture Publishing, Inc.

Quality Management: Applications for Therapeutic Recreation
      edited by Bob Riley
Recreation and Leisure: Issues in an Era of Change, Third Edition
      edited by Thomas Goodale and Peter A. Witt
The Recreation Connection to Self-Esteem—A Resource Manual for the Park, Recreation and
    Community Services Professional
      by The California Park and Recreation Society
Recreation Economic Decisions: Comparing Benefits and Costs, Second Edition
      by John B. Loomis and Richard G. Walsh
Recreation Programming and Activities for Older Adults
      by Jerold E. Elliott and Judith A. Sorg-Elliott
Recreation Programs That Work for At-Risk Youth: The Challenge of Shaping the Future
      edited by Peter A. Witt and John L. Crompton
Reference Manual for Writing Rehabilitation Therapy Treatment Plans
      by Penny Hogberg and Mary Johnson
Research in Therapeutic Recreation: Concepts and Methods
      edited by Marjorie J. Malkin and Christine Z. Howe
Risk Management in Therapeutic Recreation: A Component of Quality Assurance
      by Judith Voelkl
A Social History of Leisure Since 1600
      by Gary Cross
A Social Psychology of Leisure
      by Roger C. Mannell and Douglas A. Kleiber
The Sociology of Leisure
      by John R. Kelly and Geoffrey Godbey
Therapeutic Activity Intervention with the Elderly: Foundations and Practices
      by Barbara A. Hawkins, Marti E. May and Nancy Brattain Rogers
Therapeutic Recreation: Cases and Exercises
      by Barbara C. Wilhite and M. Jean Keller
Therapeutic Recreation in the Nursing Home
      by Linda Buettner and Shelley L. Martin
Therapeutic Recreation Protocol for Treatment of Substance Addictions
      by Rozanne W. Faulkner
Time for Life—The Surprising Ways Americans Use Their Time
      by John P. Robinson and Geoffrey Godbey
A Training Manual for Americans With Disabilities Act Compliance in Parks and Recreation
    Settings
      by Carol Stensrud
Understanding Leisure and Recreation: Mapping the Past, Charting the Future
      edited by Edgar L. Jackson and Thomas L. Burton

Venture Publishing, Inc.
1999 Cato Avenue
State College, PA 16801

Phone: (814) 234-4561; Fax: (814) 234-1651